KEY TOPICS IN
UROLOGY

M. Underwood
MD FRCS (Urol)
Glasgow Royal Infirmary,
Glasgow, UK

R. Alexander
FRCS (Urol)
Royal Alexandra Hospital,
Paisley, UK

M. Gurun
FRCS (Urol)
Ayr Hospital, Ayr, UK

G. Jones
FRCS (Urol)
Glasgow Royal Infirmary,
Glasgow, UK

Consultant Editor
D. Kirk
DM FRCS
Gartnaval General Hospital,
Glasgow, UK

© BIOS Scientific Publishers Limited, 2003

First published 2003

A CIP catalogue record for this book is available from the British Library.

ISBN 1 85996 149 5

BIOS Scientific Publishers Ltd
9 Newtec Place, Magdalen Road, Oxford OX4 1RE, UK
Tel. +44 (0)1865 726286. Fax +44 (0)1865 246823
World Wide Web home page: http://www.bios.co.uk/

Important Note from the Publisher
The information contained within this book was obtained by BIOS Scientific Publishers Ltd from sources believed by us to be reliable. However, while every effort has been made to ensure its accuracy, no responsibility for loss or injury whatsoever occasioned to any person acting or refraining from action as a result of information contained herein can be accepted by the authors or publishers.

The reader should remember that medicine is a constantly evolving science and while the authors and publishers have ensured that all dosages, applications and practices are based on current indications, there may be specific practices which differ between communities. You should always follow the guidelines laid down by the manufacturers of specific products and the relevant authorities in the country in which you are practising.

Coventry University

Production Editor: Phil Dines
Typeset by Servis Filmsetting Ltd, Manchester, UK
Printed by The Cromwell Press, Trowbridge, UK

CONTENTS

ABBREVIATIONS

ACE	angiotensin converting enzyme
AMH	anti Mullerian hormone
ATP	adenosine triphosphate
BNI	bladder neck incision
CBP	chronic bacterial prostatitis
CRP	C-reactive protein
DMSA	dimercaptosuccinic acid
DTPA	diethylenetriamepentacetic acid
EDTA	ethylenediaminetetraacetic acid
EHL	electrohydraulic lithotripsy
ESR	erythrocyte sedimentation rate
Fr size	French size
GFR	glomerular filtration rate
GI	gastrointestinal
IVU	intravenous urogram
Mag3	mercaptoacetyltriglycine
NIADDK	National Institute of Arthritis, Diabetes, Digestive and Kidney Disease
PCNL	percutaneous nephrolithotomy
PR	per rectum
PSA	prostatic specific antigen
PTH	parathyroid hormone
TENS	transcutaneous electrical nerve stimulation
TURP	transurethral resection of prostate

PREFACE

This book has been written to provide valuable information for those candidates about to sit higher surgical specialty exams where a sound urological knowledge is required.

It also will provide a reference guide for urological nurse practitioners and General Practitioners who require an up-to-date outline for diagnosis, investigation and treatment of common urological disorders.

Much of this information has been sourced from texts, specific Internet web pages, American and European urology guidelines and from the authors' own clinical and operative experiences.

ACUTE AND CHRONIC PROSTATITIS

Acute prostatitis is a condition caused by inflammation and/or infection and is classified as bacterial or non-bacterial. Causative organisms include Gram-negative organisms, most commonly *Escherichia coli*, *Proteus* spp., *Klebsiella* spp. and *Pseudomonas* spp.

Clinical features

Acute prostatitis is an acute severe systemic illness. Patients present with symptoms of a urinary tract infection: dysuria, frequency and urgency. Patients may also experience low back pain, perineal, penile and sometimes rectal pain. Clinical examination reveals signs localized to the prostate: extremely tender, swollen and tense. Signs of bacteraemia, pyrexia and tachycardia may also be present. Patients with acute prostatitis may present with acute retention secondary to prostatic oedema.

Diagnosis

A mid-stream urine sample for dipstick testing, culture for bacteria and antibiotic sensitivity is obtained and blood cultures for bacteria and antibiotic sensitivity. Serum PSA may also be raised.

Management

Adequate hydration should be maintained, rest encouraged and analgesics such as non-steroidal anti-inflammatory drugs used.

As acute prostatitis is a serious and severe illness empirical therapy should be started immediately. Parenteral or oral treatment should be selected according to the clinical condition of the patient. If there is deterioration or failure to respond to oral therapy urgent admission and parenteral therapy should be arranged.

For patients requiring parenteral therapy antibiotics covering the likely organisms should be used. A high-dose broad spectrum cephalosporin, for example, cefuroxime, cefotaxime or ceftriaxone plus gentamycin, is appropriate. When clinically improved the therapy can be switched to oral treatment according to sensitivities.

For patients suitable for oral therapy, quinolones can be used: ciprofloxacin 500 mg twice daily for 28 days.

If the patient fails to respond fully to therapy the diagnosis of a prostatic abscess should be considered. This can be confirmed by transrectal ultrasound scan or computed tomography scan of the prostate gland. If present perineal or transurethral drainage will be necessary. If acute prostatitis is managed correctly the prognosis is good and cure likely. At least 4 weeks of antibiotic therapy is recommended in all patients to try to prevent chronic bacterial prostatitis.

When the patient has recovered his urinary tract should be investigated to exclude a structural cause for urinary tract infection.

Chronic prostatitis

By use of the lower urinary tract quantitative localization procedure (The Stamey Test), chronic prostatitis can be differentiated into:

1. Chronic bacterial prostatitis (CBP).
2. Chronic abacterial prostatitis/chronic pelvic pain syndrome–inflammatory (CAP/CPPS). This was previously called chronic non-bacterial prostatitis.
3. Chronic abacterial prostatitis/chronic pelvic pain syndrome–non-inflammatory (CAP/CPPS). This was previously called prostatodynia.

Many experts believe that CAP/CPPS inflammatory and non-inflammatory are variables of one condition. This area is currently being extensively researched. At present the National Institutes of Health classification includes the two conditions both separately and grouped together.

Bacterial prostatitis (acute or chronic) is uncommon compared with CAP.

Chronic bacterial prostatitis

CBP is characterized by the recovery of pathogenic bacteria, in significant numbers, from prostatic fluid in the absence of concomitant urinary infection. Usual causative bacteria are those causing acute bacterial prostatitis, most commonly *E. coli*.

Some Gram-positive organisms such as *Staphylococcus aureus*, *Streptococcus faecalis* and enterococci cause CBP. The role of other Gram-positive organisms such as coagulase negative staphylococci, non-group D streptococci and diphtheroids remains controversial and subject to much debate.

Chronic abacterial prostatitis – inflammatory and non-inflammatory

The aetiology of these conditions is unknown. Although pathogenic bacteria are rarely found a significant number of patients appear to respond to antibiotics. This does not prove the condition is caused by bacteria as most of the studies had no control group and some antibiotics have anti-inflammatory effects.

There is evidence that CAP/CPPS is caused by some form of persistent antigen within the prostate gland. This antigen may be an organism/remnant or could be a constituent of urine which has refluxed into the gland.

Urodynamic and cystoscopic examinations on patients with CAP/CPPS–non-inflammatory have led to suggestions that symptoms may be caused by functional urethral obstruction, pelvic sympathetic nervous system dysfunction and interstitial cystitis. These remain unproved.

Whatever the aetiology of chronic prostatitis it undoubtedly has a very significant physical and psychological impact.

Clinical features

Chronic prostatitis has no standardized clinical definition despite being well recognized in clinical practice. It is characterized by a variety of symptoms most of which involve genital pain. These include:

1. Perineal pain.
2. Lower abdominal pain.
3. Penile pain (especially penile tip).
4. Testicular pain.
5. Ejaculatory discomfort or pain.
6. Rectal and lower back pain.
7. Dysuria.

Attempts have been made to evaluate the symptoms of chronic prostatitis and reports suggest the first five symptoms listed above are more discriminatory. Strictly, symptoms should have been present for at least 6 months to diagnose chronic prostatitis although in practice the diagnosis is made after a shorter duration of symptoms. There are few objective clinical signs and the prostate gland may, or may not, be locally or diffusely tender to palpation. There is also no evidence that the different types of chronic prostatitis can be differentiated on the basis of symptoms and signs.

Diagnosis

The investigation of chronic prostatitis which has been the standard for evidence based research is the lower urinary tract localization procedure (Stamey Test). Although time consuming this is the most accurate method for differentiating CBP, CAP/CPPS–inflammatory and CAP/CPPS–non-inflammatory.

1. The Stamey Test.

1. The foreskin should be fully retracted and the penis well cleaned to prevent contamination.
2. A 5–10 ml sample of first-void urethral urine (VB1) should be collected.
3. The patient should urinate a further 100–200 ml urine and then a further 5–10 ml sample of mid-stream bladder urine (VB2) should be collected.
4. By digital rectal examination a vigorous massage of the prostate gland should be performed for 1 min, from periphery towards the midline with a sterile container held over the glans to collect any expressed prostatic secretions (EPS).
5. A wet preparation microscopic examination of a sample of expressed prostatic secretions should be made to determine the number of polymorphonuclear leucocytes (PMNL) per high power field ($\times 400$).
6. Immediately after the massage another 5–10 ml post-massage urine (VB3) should be collected.
7. All three urine samples should have microscopy and quantitative culture.

A dry prostatic massage is reasonably common.

Interpretation of results

- To assign an organism to the prostate the colony count in the EPS and VB3 is required to be at least 10 times greater than in VB1–2.
- For prostatic inflammation ≥ 10 PMNL/high power field (hpf) is considered diagnostic. In cases of a dry expressate a PMNL count of 10/hpf greater in VB3 than VB1 and VB2 is diagnostic of prostatitis.
- If there is significant bacteriuria in both VB2 and VB3 3 days of nitrofurantoin 50 mg four times daily, which is not prostate penetrating, should be given and the procedure then repeated.
- An EPS pH ≥ 8 suggests prostatitis although it is not diagnostic.
- Clumping of PMNL and presence of lipid laden macrophages suggests prostatitis, although not diagnostic.

Management

Patients should be given a detailed explanation of their condition with particular emphasis on the long-term implications for their health. This should be reinforced by giving them clear and accurate written information.

Chronic bacterial prostatitis

Many antimicrobials penetrate the prostate gland poorly. In CBP the gland is either subacutely inflamed or non-inflamed.

Treatment should be chosen according to antimicrobial sensitivities.

1. Recommended regimens. For patients with CBP first-line treatment is with a quinolone such as ciprofloxacin 500 mg twice daily for 28 days or ofloxacin 200 mg twice daily for 28 days.

Prostatic calculi have been suggested as a source for recurrent infection. They are extremely common radiographically. Radical transurethral prostatectomy or total prostatectomy is effective in some patients if they are selected carefully.

Chronic abacterial prostatitis/chronic pelvic pain syndrome

There are no universally effective treatments for CAP/CPPS. The lack of knowledge of the aetiology of these conditions means that no specific recommendations can be made and treatment choice is usually trial and error. There is currently a systematic review of therapies for CAP/CPPS taking place.

Despite negative cultures most clinicians try antibiotics initially to cover occult infection. This may be effective in a number of patients although this does not mean that the problem was genuinely infective. Treatment is as for CBP with a quinolone or tetracycine.

Other treatments include:

1. Transurethral microwave thermatherapy (CAP/CPPS–inflammatory).
2. α-blockers:
   (i) Terazosin 2–10 mg for 28 days. The dose should be increased gradually according to symptomatic response (CAP/CPPS–inflammatory and non-inflammatory).
   (ii) Alfuzosin 2.5 mg three times daily for 42 days in patients with confirmed urodynamic abnormalities.
3. Non-steroidal anti-inflammatory drugs (CAP/CPPS–inflammatory).
4. Cernilton (pollen extract) probably acts as an anti-inflammatory. One tablet three times daily for 6 months (CAP/CPPS).
5. The bioflavonoid, quercetin 500 mg twice daily for 28 days (CAP/CPPS–inflammatory and non-inflammatory).
6. Stress management. No specific therapy has been tested or advocated although referral for psychological assessment may be appropriate in some. Diazepam 5 mg twice daily for 90 days has produced symptomatic benefit although benzodiazepines are not recommended in clinical practice because of dependency.

Further reading

Stamey TA. Bacteriologic localisation patterns in bacterial prostatitis and urethritis. *Invest Urol*, 1968; **5**: 492–518.

Nickel JC. Prostatitis: myths and realities. *Urology*, 1998; **51**: 362–366.

ACUTE PYELONEPHRITIS

Definition

Inflammation of the kidney and the renal pelvis.

Clinical presentation

There is a clinical spectrum which may range from cystitis with some mild flank pain to Gram-negative septicaemia. Classical description is of sudden onset of fever associated with loin pain and tenderness. Approximately 75% of patients give a history of lower urinary tract infection. Associated nausea and vomiting are frequently present.

Examination

Most patients show signs of fever and exhibit loin tenderness on palpation.

Investigations

1. Urine culture. Twenty percent will have negative Gram stains because they have less than 100 000 cfu/ml. Urine microscopy will normally reveal pus cells and red blood cells. Common organisms cultured are:

- *E. coli* 80%.
- *Proteus.*
- *Klebsiella.*
- *Enterobacter.*

2. Blood tests

- White cell count normally raised.
- C-reactive protein elevated.
- Creatinine levels may be elevated.
- Blood cultures may be positive.

3. Radiology. Imaging is important in the acute phase to differentiate between acute pyelonephritis and an obstructed infected kidney in those patients who are unwell.

4. Intravenous urogram appearances. This may show:

- Generalized renal enlargement.
- Focal renal enlargement, mimicking an intra-renal mass, may be present and is described as acute lobar nephronia. It must be distinguished from a true intra-renal mass or an intra-renal abscess.
- Delayed excretion on affected side. This is thought due to obstruction of renal tubules due to parenchymal oedema and local vasoconstriction.
- Dilatation of renal pelvis and ureter. This is thought due to local effects of bacterial endotoxin impairing ureteric peristalsis.

5. Ultrasound scan. This may show:

- Renal enlargement.
- Collecting system dilatation.
- Focal nephritis (lobar nephronia).

However, it is not unusual for both IVU and USS to be normal reinforcing the point that acute pyelonephritis is essentially a clinical diagnosis.

Management

Many patients can be managed at home and do not require hospitalization. The mainstays of therapy are identical whether in a hospital or home setting.

1. Antibiotics. Appropriate antibiotics are:

- Co-amoxiclav.
- Aminoglycosides.
- Quinolones.

2. Fluids. Fluid levels are achieved either by encouraging extra oral intake or by intravenous administration.

Patients should be warned that they are likely to have persistent fever and flank pain for 2–3 days after the institution of appropriate antibiotic therapy.

Persistence of symptoms beyond 72 h should raise the concern of developing perinephric or intrarenal abscess.

Duration of antibiotic therapy should be for 14 days. Approximately 10–30% of patients relapse after completing their 14-day course. The vast majority of these respond to a second 14-day course.

Sequelae

Patients can go on to develop a perinephric or renal abscess and some will go on to develop chronic pyelonephritis.

Further reading

McRae SN, Dairiki Shortliffe LM. Bacterial infections of the genitourinary tract. In: Tanagho EA, McAninch JW, eds. *Smith's General Urology*, 15th ed. Ohio: McGraw-Hill Education, 2000; 237–264.

ACUTE RENAL FAILURE (ARF)

Acute renal failure (ARF) is the generic term used to define an abrupt decrease in renal function sufficient to result in retention of nitrogenous wastes in the body. The hallmark of ARF is progressive azotaemia caused by the accumulation of the nitrogenous end-products of metabolism. This accumulation is accompanied by a wide range of other disturbances depending on the severity and duration of the renal dysfunction. These include metabolic derangements such as metabolic acidosis and hyperkalaemia, disturbances of body fluid balance and effects on many other organ systems.

Causes

The various aetiologies of ARF can be grouped into three major categories:

1. Decreased renal blood flow (pre-renal).
2. A renal parenchymal insult (intra-renal).
3. Obstructed urine flow (post-renal or obstructive).

Identification of either a pre-renal or post-renal cause of ARF makes the initiation of a specific therapy possible. If, however, these two categories can be ruled out, then a parenchymal cause can be implicated. The renal parenchymal causes of ARF are usually subdivided into those primarily affecting the glomeruli, the intra-renal vasculature or the renal interstitium. The term 'acute tubular necrosis' (ATN) denotes another broad category of intrinsic renal failure that cannot be attributed to glomerular, vascular, or interstitial causes.

Pre-renal causes of acute renal failure

Result from a decrease in renal blood flow. The glomerular filtration rate (GFR) is reduced and the kidney retains water and salt, causing oliguria, production of a concentrated urine, and a progressive inability to excrete nitrogenous wastes.

Intra-renal acute renal failure

1. *Glomerular disease.* Most of the glomerular diseases producing ARF are felt to be immunologically mediated and result in disrupted glomerular filtration. Progression of the inflammatory process leads to destruction of glomerulus and a decrease in the GFR.

2. *ATN.* The exact cause of this is not clear.

3. *Interstitial disease.* Interstitial nephritis is a complex collection of disease processes with a poorly understood pathophysiology. An inflammatory process is initiated in the renal interstitium in response to a wide variety of stimuli (toxic, metabolic, infectious, immune, infiltrative), although drugs are probably the most common causes.

Post-renal acute renal failure

A simple mechanical or functional obstruction to the free flow of urine precludes its excretion, producing renal failure.

1. Acute tubular necrosis. The characteristic tubular injury in this disorder represents a non-specific response that can be seen with a variety of renal insults, including renal ischaemia and exposure to exogenous or endogenous nephrotoxins. The net effect is a rapid decline in renal function that may require a period of dialysis before spontaneous resolution occurs.

There are two major histologic changes that take place in ATN:

1. Tubular necrosis with sloughing of the epithelial cells.
2. Occlusion of the tubular lumina by casts and by cellular debris.

These changes may be patchy and seem mild compared with the degree of the renal failure. In addition to the tubular obstruction, two other factors appear to contribute to the development of renal failure in ATN: backleak of filtrate across the damaged tubular epithelia and a primary reduction in glomerular filtration. The decrease in glomerular filtration results both from arteriolar vasoconstriction and from mesangial contraction.

The decline in renal function in ATN has a variable onset. It typically begins abruptly following a hypotensive episode, rhabdomyolysis, or the administration of a radiocontrast media. In comparison, when aminoglycosides are the cause, the onset is more insidious, with the first rise in creatinine being at 7 days or more.

Diagnosis

1. History and physical examination. Often, the history alone can suggest the cause as being pre-renal, renal, or post-renal. Physical examination is usually most helpful in assessing the volume status of a patient. Both the total volume and the effective circulating volume must be considered. Clues for the presence of a systemic disease (e.g. vasculitis, chronic heart failure, liver disease) should be sought. Despite a careful history and physical examination, the aetiology of ARF often remains unclear and additional tests must be carried out.

2. Examination of the urine. A dipstick positive for protein (3+) suggests intrinsic renal disease with glomerular damage. Pre-renal failure, obstruction and acute tubular necrosis tend to be associated with less proteinurea (trace–1+) than a glomerular lesion. If there is proteinurea present it should be quantified using a 24-h urine collection. If there is greater than 3 g of protein, a glomerular, rather than a vascular or interstitial, process is more likely.

A dipstick positive for blood indicates the presence of red blood cells (RBCs) (>5/HPF). If no RBCs are present, then there may be either myoglobin or haemoglobin present in the urine.

In most cases the most significant amount of information comes from the examination of the sediment of a centrifuged urine sample. The urine is scanned under high power for RBCs, white cells, renal tubular epithelial cells, oval fat bodies, bacteria and crystals.

Casts are formed from urinary Tamm–Horsfall protein, which is a product of the tubular epithelial cells. This protein tends to gel in conditions of high concentration and when mixed with red cells, tubular cells or cellular debris. Thus, the composition of this cast reflects the contents of the tubule. Hyaline casts are those that are devoid of contents, and are seen with dehydration, after exercise, or in association with glomerular proteinuria. Red cell casts indicate glomerular haematuria, as seen with glomerulonephritis. White cell casts imply the presence of renal parenchymal inflammation. Granular casts are composed of cellular remnants and debris. Fatty casts are usually associated with heavy proteinuria and the nephrotic syndrome (although they can be present in other non-glomerular disease).

In patients with pre-renal failure, the sediment usually lacks cells, casts and cellular debris. Similarly, post-renal causes of ARF tend to be associated with a benign sediment. The presence of RBCs and red cell casts is characteristic of a glomerular lesion. WBCs and white cell casts are seen in acute interstitial nephritis.

3. Serum and urine chemical analysis. Creatinine is formed from the breakdown of muscle creatinine and is proportional to the muscle mass. It should be stable from day to day. The creatinine concentration is a function of the amount of creatinine entering the blood from muscle, its volume of distribution, and its rate of excretion. Since the first two are usually constant, changes in the serum creatinine level would usually be a result of a change in the GFR. Abrupt cessation of glomerular filtration causes the serum creatinine to rise by 1–3 mg/dl daily. The blood urea also rises with renal dysfunction, but is influenced by extra-renal factors as well. Increased protein intake, catabolism, GI bleeding and many other factors will affect blood urea.

An important point to remember about elevations of serum creatinine and urea is that they are late signs of renal dysfunction because GFR may need to be reduced by as much as 75% before elevations reach abnormal amounts. Generally, a serum urea to creatinine ratio of greater than 20 suggests pre-renal failure rather than ATN, which is associated with a level of 10 to 1. This value is subject to significant variation.

4. Urine osmolality. Normally, the kidney can concentrate urine to levels greater than 1200 mOsm/kg. The ability to do this depends on an intact tubular system. Serum osmolality levels greater than 500 mOsm/kg suggest pre-renal failure. By comparison, extensive tubular damage, such as that seen in ATN, impairs the ability of the kidney to generate a concentrated urine. Typically, in ATN the urine osmolality is approximately 300–350, which is similar to the serum osmolality.

5. Urine sodium concentration. Urine sodium excretion reflects how well the nephron retains the filtered sodium load. With renal hypoperfusion, due to either volume depletion or ineffective circulation, if tubule function is maintained, the kidney will avidly retain sodium as a result of increased proximal and distal reabsorption. If the kidney is responding appropriately to a decreased effective intravascular volume, urine sodium concentration will usually be low (less than 20 mEq/l).

6. Radiology. Intravenous pyelogram (IVP) provides an anatomic picture of the kidney but does not facilitate the evaluation of kidney function. It also subjects the patient to a dye load, which can potentially be harmful to kidneys that may have already suffered previous insult.

Renal ultrasound is the most valuable diagnostic technique for the assessment of the patient with ARF. It can be performed easily in the patient with impaired renal function and has no associated morbidity. It is a sensitive test for obstruction (93–98%) and provides information about kidney size (the kidney size can be helpful in judging the chronicity of the kidney disease).

Computed tomography (CT) can be helpful in some patients. Hydronephrosis can be recognized without contrast. The cause of obstruction (e.g. lymphoma, retroperitoneal fibrosis) can often be delineated. CT is the technique of choice for visualizing ureteral obstruction at the level of the bony pelvis.

Radionuclide scans can be used if there is a concern about vascular perfusion of the kidneys. Percutaneous nephrostomy combined with antegrade pyelography can be employed to diagnose the precise level of obstruction in the urinary tract. Ultimately, if the diagnosis is still unclear, the patient may need a renal biopsy.

Specific diseases causing acute renal failure

1. *Pre-renal disease.* A reduction in renal blood flow is the most common cause of acute renal failure. This can occur from true volume depletion or from selective renal ischaemia (as in bilateral renal artery stenosis). The usual causes of pre-renal failure are true volume depletion, advanced liver disease, and congestive heart failure.

- Pre-renal failure caused by true volume depletion. The cause of volume depletion is usually evident from the history and examination. In severe cases the patient may be in hypovolaemic shock. Oliguria is present in most individuals and this is an appropriate response given the clinical situation. Normal or increased urine output indicates that an osmotic agent or other diuretic agent is acting, or that there is tubular dysfunction such as ATN.
- Pre-renal failure caused by advanced liver disease. Liver disease is associated with two major changes in renal function: sodium retention, initially manifested as ascites, and a progressive decline in GFR. Both humoral and haemodynamic factors play a primary role in the development of these problems. The progressive decline in renal function that occurs in hepatic cirrhosis is thought to be haemodynamically mediated because tubular function is intact (as evidenced by low urine sodium concentration and a normal urinalysis) and the kidneys are histologically intact.
- Pre-renal failure caused by congestive heart failure (CHF) is associated with two major alterations in renal function: sodium retention early in the course of the disease and a decline in GFR as cardiac function worsens. Neurohumoral factors and certain therapies may contribute to these problems.

Complications of acute renal failure

1. *Cardiovascular system.* In the oliguric patient with ARF, volume overload, oedema and pulmonary congestion is an ever-present threat. Pericarditis may rarely complicate the course of ARF, and may occur at relatively low serum creatinine levels accompanying the hepatorenal syndrome. Pericarditis can lead to tamponade.

2. *Pulmonary system complications.* Pulmonary infiltrates due to oedema from volume overload and/or infection are encountered frequently in ARF. The development of pulmonary complications in ARF is an adverse prognostic factor.

3. *Gastrointestinal system complications.* The most common GI manifestations of ARF are severe nausea, vomiting, and anorexia. Upper GI bleeding is another significant complication. Stress ulcers and gastritis are common.

4. *Neurologic system complications.* CNS disorders are frequent accompaniments of ARF. Initially, lethargy, somnolence, lassitude and fatigue are present.

These symptoms may progress to irritability, confusion, disorientation, decreased memory, twitching and myoclonus. In advanced cases, generalized seizures may occur with somnolence and coma.

The encephalopathy of ARF has not yet been firmly identified as a complication of a single specific identifiable toxin. Thus, the pathophysiology of neurologic complications of ARF remains unclear.

5. Infectious complications. ARF and infections are commonly associated. Not only is septicaemia frequently associated with the onset of ARF, but also infections often complicate the course of ARF. Common sites are pulmonary, urinary and peritonitis. These infectious complications can be a leading source of morbidity and mortality.

6. Endocrine system complications. Several hormonal abnormalities have been described in ARF. For example, ATN is often associated with disturbances in divalent ion metabolism (hypocalcaemia, hyperphosphataemia and hypermagnesaemia). Altered PTH action and vitamin D metabolism may play a pathogenic role in the hypocalcaemia and hyperphosphataemia.

High plasma renin activity and angiotensin II levels often occur in the setting of ARF. Whether these agents contribute to the hypertension has yet to be determined.

7. Disorders of electrolyte metabolism. Hyperkalaemia, hyponatraemia, metabolic acidosis and hyperuricaemia often occur in ARF.

Treatment of acute renal failure

1. Resuscitation. The two most common causes of death early in the resuscitative phase are hyperkalaemia and pulmonary oedema. Over-hydration with resultant pulmonary oedema is usually the iatrogenic consequence of futile attempts to restore urine output before the aetiology of the renal failure has been established. At the same time that the patient is being hydrated and metabolic/electrolyte are being managed, the aetiology of the ARF needs to be established so that the needed interventions can begin.

2. Post-renal failure. In those with post-renal failure, a passage for the drainage of urine must be created. The exact method that is used will depend entirely on the level of the obstruction and may be as simple as a urinary catheter, or as complex as a percutaneous nephrostomy tube.

3. Pre-renal failure

- Treatment for true volume depletion. Therapy for this type of ARF is aimed at restoration of the normal circulating blood volume. Fluid replacement usually depends on the clinical status of the patient. Initially, fluid boluses may be needed, and if indicated, blood transfusion may be required. The patient must be constantly reassessed to ensure that they do not become over-hydrated. The adequacy of fluid repletion can be assessed from physical examination and by monitoring renal function and urine output.

- Treatment for ARF due to advanced liver disease. Dietary sodium restriction and periods of bed rest are the mainstays of non-medical therapy in this disease entity. Medical therapies are as follows:

Diuretics therapy is often indicated and the preferred agent is spironolactone. Normally this is a fairly weak diuretic; however in cases of liver failure it is very effective. Spironolactone is the only diuretic that does not require secretion into the lumen of the kidney. Rather, it enters the collecting tubule cells from the blood side and competes for the aldosterone receptor. The rate of diuresis needs to be slow and steady.

Paracentesis may be helpful in those patients with tense ascites. Albumen may be given at the same time to help prevent the worsening of intravascular depletion. A peritoneovenous shunt may be used, draining ascitic fluid from the internal jugular vein into the vascular space. The side effects are often severe.

- Treatment of ARF caused by congestive heart failure. The use of diuretics may be of some help as this will increase the renal output. Another option is a trial of iatrogenic agents to help increase cardiac output and thus increase renal perfusion. ACE inhibitors may also be helpful.

Further reading

Abuelo GJ. *Renal Failure: Diagnosis and Treatment*. The Netherlands: Kluwer Academic Publishers, 1995.

BASIC MOLECULAR BIOLOGY OF UROLOGICAL CANCERS

Introduction

Molecular diagnostic and prognostic markers for specific urological conditions will become an important tool for future clinical practice. This chapter will focus on the background to this subject and highlight specific examples in tumour biology.

The aberration of the genome as being responsible for the origins of cancer has been known for many years but until only recently has the involvement of specific genes been demonstrated at the molecular level. Three broad classes of genes appear to be involved in the transition of a normal cell to a malignant one. The first are oncogenes – genes related to normal cellular genes whose aberrant expression contributes to malignancy. The second class of genes are the tumour suppressor genes, which normally act to control cell proliferation and whose loss or inactivation is again associated with tumourigenesis. Thirdly, there is a class of genes involved in DNA repair (mutator genes) which, when mutated, predispose the patient to developing cancer.

Oncogenes

Oncogenes are involved in the basic essential functions of the cell related to cell growth and differentiation. The products of these genes are detected at many different cellular locations and mutation or an increase in the gene copy number (amplification) in any one of these genes may disrupt the response of the cell to signals which control its growth These genes are located at four specific sites. The first group encode proteins capable of autocrine stimulation, that is, SIS. A second group the growth factor receptors, that is, epidermal growth factor receptor EGFR or c-erbB. The third group comprise the signal transducers – the three main members of the RAS family HRAS, KRAS, NRAS. These genes encode for a protein p21, which can bind GTP and exhibits GTPase activity. The final group of oncogenes are involved in the control of gene expression by their action on DNA itself, that is, MYC, FOS and JUN.

Tumour suppressor genes

These genes are involved in cellular growth. Each dividing cell progresses through a specific cycle of events and 'checkpoints' throughout this cell cycle ensure that this mechanism proceeds through DNA synthesis, growth and mitosis. Many tumour suppressor genes act at these checkpoints and these specific genes have been termed guardians or policemen of the genome. Retinoblastoma gene on 13q (RB1) and p53 on 17p are known to bind to DNA and have been shown to act at specific sites of the cell cycle. Their function appears to be as negative cell regulators of growth by controlling transcription of cell cycle dependent genes. Once mutated in tumours they can no longer regulate their target genes, leading to uncontrolled proliferation with aberrant differentiation and eventual tumour formation.

DNA repair genes (mutator genes)

This group of genes are involved in DNA repair, which, when mutated, predispose the patient to developing cancer. These genes were discovered during studies of hereditary non-polyposis colorectal cancer. The first mutator gene MSH-2 was found to have a strong homology with the MUT-2 gene occurring in bacteria and isolated on the short arm of chromosome 2. A second gene concerned with DNA repair is MLH-1 which is located on the short arm of chromosome 3.

Any combination of these changes may be found in an individual tumour. The overall progression to malignancy therefore is a complex and sometimes multistage event.

Bladder cancer

Our current understanding of the genetics of bladder cancer recurrence and disease progression appears to be secondary to two distinct genetic pathways. The first is characterized by alterations to chromosome 9 and the latter to abnormal p53 function.

In most low-grade transitional cell carcinomas (TCC), partial or complete loss of chromosome 9 is the only genetic aberration. Four candidate tumour suppressor genes (TSGs) have been mapped to chromosome 9; 9p21 is a common region of deletion shared by many carcinomas including bladder and this region contains the genes p15, p16 and p19^{ARF}.

The alternative pathway to progression appears to be due to aberrant p53. Deletion frequencies of p53 can be as high as 70% in bladder tumours of high grade/stage. This gene has been widely studied and mutations show a close correlation with progression to muscle invasion and poor clinical outcome.

There is, however, involvement of many other genetic aberrations in these pathways. Amplification and overexpression of the oncogene c-erbB2 (located at 17q21) has been correlated with a poor clinical outcome in bladder cancer. In addition, advanced bladder cancer stage/grade has been correlated with deletion of 3p14 and increased copy number of chromosome 7.

This brief outline serves to illustrate the complex genetics of bladder cancer recurrence and progression.

Prostate cancer

Despite the substantial clinical importance of prostate cancer, the molecular mechanisms underlying the development and progression of the disease are poorly understood. The aim of molecular genetics is to reveal the genetic alterations and genes that are involved in disease processes. Linkage analysis implicated chromosomal loci that may harbour prostate cancer susceptibility genes. These analyses have indicated that losses of chromosomes 6q, 8p, 10q, 13q and 16q, as well as gains of 7, 8q and Xq are particularly common in prostate cancer. There is also a strong evidence that genes, such as androgen receptor gene (AR), e-cadherin and PTEN, are involved in the development and progression of prostate cancer.

Treatment of advanced prostate cancer aims at inhibiting cancer growth by suppression of endogenous androgen action or production. The transition from hormone dependent to hormone independent tumour genesis is assumed to be a cascade of genetic alterations caused by activation of oncogenes and/or inactivation of tumour suppressor genes. For example high levels of the proto-oncogene bcl 2 have been associated with androgen independent prostate cancer. Two novel candidate oncogenes (PTI-1 and HPC1) have been reported to be involved in prostate cancer. The PTI-1 gene, prostate tumour inducing gene 1, was shown to be expressed in prostate cancer and not in normal prostate tissue. The HPC1 gene hereditary prostate cancer gene 1 is probably involved in the familial form of prostate cancer and is localized on the long arm of chromosome 1. The function of both genes and their encoded proteins is not known. The involvement of genetic changes in tumour suppressor genes (e.g. retinoblastoma gene and the p53 gene) in prostate cancer have been documented. However, the role of p53 mutations in prostate cancer is still uncertain. Recently, three novel candidate tumour suppressor genes (Mxil, maspin and KA 11) have been reported to be involved in prostate cancer. Msil, a suspected repressor of the c-myc oncogene, has been reported to be mutated in 40% of primary prostate tumours. Maspin was shown to inhibit prostatic cancer motility and invasion. KA11 was shown to have metastasis suppressing activity in prostate cancer and is localized on chromosome 11p11.2.

Renal cancer

There have been significant advances in our understanding of the genetic basis of renal cancer. In particular, research in the last 5 years has demonstrated a central role for the inactivation of the von Hippel–Lindau gene (3p) by mutation or hyper-methylation in the formation of the conventional type of renal cell carcinoma. The von Hippel–Lindau syndrome is characterized by germ-line inactivating mutation whereas sporadic renal carcinoma is associated with somatic mutations. Another form of familial renal cancer, the hereditary papillary renal cell carcinoma, has been shown to be consequent upon activating mutations of the c-met proto-oncogene.

Testes cancer

Cytogenetic abnormalities in testicular tumours are beginning to be explored. Detailed karyotypic analysis has revealed non-random changes in chromosomes 1, 5, 6, 7, 9, 11, 12, 16, 17, 21, 22 and X. Of these, a duplication on the short arm of chromosome 12p, or isochromosome i(12p), is the best studied and the most characteristic. This marker was present in one or more copies in approximately 89% of seminomas and 81% of non-seminomas studied. Most of the remaining patients had other abnormalities involving the 12p chromosome. The i(12p) marker is also observed in extra-gonadal germ-cell tumours and occasionally in ovarian dysgerminomas but is rare in other tumours. It is a highly specific marker for germ-cell tumours and a useful diagnostic tool in cancers of unknown origin.

How i(12p) participates in the development of testis cancer is unknown. The oncogene c-ki-ras 2 resides on the short arm of chromosome 12, but amplification of this gene as a transforming event has been difficult to show. Other oncogenes and their products have been investigated, but as yet their significance and roles in the pathogenesis of testis cancer remain to be demonstrated.

Further reading

McDonald F, Ford CHJ. *Molecular Biology of Cancer*. BIOS Scientific Publishers. 1996; 1–35.

BENIGN PROSTATIC HYPERPLASIA

Benign prostatic hyperplasia (BPH) occurs histologically in approximately 75% of men over 70 years of age and men have a lifetime risk of 10–30% of having a prostatectomy. The introduction of specific medication for patients with lower urinary tract symptoms consistent with bladder outlet obstruction has changed the approach to treatment and management of patients with BPH. The prostate is located at the base of the bladder and the benign enlargement of the central and transitional zones which surround the urethra cause obstruction. The peripheral zone (which harbours 70% of prostatic carcinomas) is compressed as the prostate enlarges. The reasons for enlargement are currently unknown.

Presentation

Approximately 50% of men over the age of 50 seek help for troublesome lower urinary tract symptoms. These symptoms may be divided into irritative/storage (frequency, urgency, urge incontinence) symptoms and obstructive/voiding (poor flow, hesitancy, incomplete voiding) symptoms.

Investigations

It is important to realize that not all men with lower urinary tract symptoms have bladder outlet obstruction due to benign prostatic hyperplasia. The history and examination play an integral part of determining the diagnosis.

Patients can be assessed at specific 'one-stop' prostate assessment clinics.

A full history and completion of an International Prostate Symptom Score (IPSS) will enable the clinician to assess symptoms and impact on the quality of life. Frequency/volume charts are also of importance as these can document day and night voiding and episodes of incontinence.

A full clinical examination is mandatory. Abdominal examination may detect the presence of a palpable bladder and a rectal examination may indicate a prostatic carcinoma. Examination of the genitalia is required to exclude a phimosis.

Laboratory and clinic investigations include:

1. Mid-stream specimen of urine (MSSU).
2. Renal function.
3. Prostatic specific antigen (PSA) in selected patients (see chapter on prostatic carcinoma).
4. Flow studies and residual urine.

Management

Treatment is dependent on the patient's wishes, severity of symptoms and degree of obstruction. The indications for treatment include acute retention, recurrent urinary tract infection and severe symptoms.

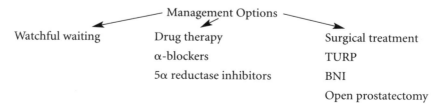

Watchful waiting	Drug therapy	Surgical treatment
	α-blockers	TURP
	5α reductase inhibitors	BNI
		Open prostatectomy

Before implementing treatment an objective measurement of maximum flow rate and ultrasound urine residual is essential. A flow rate of less than 10 ml/s will normally indicate obstruction in 90% of patients. Patients with flow studies of greater than 10 ml/s have a 1 in 3 chance of not being obstructed and therefore may not benefit from treatment for bladder outlet obstruction.

Patients can be offered conservative treatment in the form of watchful waiting as a number of clinical trials have revealed a placebo benefit (up to 25% in some series). Advice can also be given on fluid intake, bladder retraining and the appropriate use of diuretics in patients with nocturnal polyuria and congestive cardiac failure.

Drug treatments now constitute the main therapy for lower urinary tract symptoms consistent with bladder outlet obstruction.

α_1-blockers

The α receptors are found throughout the lower urinary tract but are most abundant on the trigone of the bladder and the fibromuscular stroma of the bladder neck and prostatic urethra. Relaxation of these receptors through their action on smooth muscle causes an improvement in flow rates, residual urines and symptom scores.

5αR Inhibitors

These drugs work by blocking the conversion of testosterone to the active metabolite dihydrotestosterone. The medication causes a reduction in prostatic volume of up to 25% over 3 months. The treatment needs to be maintained for the benefit to continue. It is only appropriate in larger prostates (>30 g, PSA>3 ng/ml).

Surgery

Transurethral resection of the prostate (TURP) involves endoscopic resection of the hyperplastic tissue surrounding the urethra. The best outcomes for surgery are when patients have proven obstruction with urodynamic pressure flow studies or a flow rate of <10 ml/s. Transurethral surgery can result in incontinence from sphincter damage (1%), erectile dysfunction and retrograde ejaculation.

A bladder neck incision (BNI) may be performed in the presence of a tight prostate/bladder neck without enlargement of the prostate.

Open surgery is still performed for large glands (>100–150 g). This may be performed either by a retropubic or transvesical route.

Other treatments are presently being evaluated, including ablation by laser treatment, thermotherapy and high temperature radio frequency. To date none of these have proved effective long term when compared with the 'gold standard' TURP.

Further reading

Shapiro E. Pathophysiology of clinical benign prostatic hyperplasia. *Urol Clin N Am*, 1995; **22**: 285–290.

BENIGN TUMOURS OF THE KIDNEY

Before the use of CT and ultrasound scanning in urological practice, benign tumours of the kidney were infrequently detected because they rarely caused symptoms or morbidity. The different types of benign renal tumour are outlined below.

Epithelial tumours

1. Cortical adenoma. Cortical adenomas are small well-defined tumours, which do not cause symptoms during life and are found commonly at autopsy in people over 40 years, the vast majority of whom are males. They form pale yellow to grey subcapsular, cortical masses usually less than 2 cm in diameter.

Histologically, most cortical adenomas show complex, branching papillary fronds that project into and fill a cystic space. Less often they form closely packed tubules or cords. The cells are uniform and small and usually lack cytologic features of malignancy. Occasionally they may be large with eosinophilic or clear cytoplasm.

Adenomas less than 3 cm in diameter rarely metastasize and the smaller the tumour, the more unlikely it is to metastasize. On the other hand larger tumours metastasize at a frequency that appears to be a linear function of their diameter. The dilemma is that all cancers begin as small lesions and no histologic criteria have been found, as yet, to distinguish a small carcinoma from an adenoma. Currently, the separation is based predominantly on the size of the lesion. Tumours less than 3 cm are called adenomas and larger ones are called carcinomas.

2. Renal oncocytoma. These are almost always found incidentally and, unlike cortical adenomas, have a gross appearance that differs markedly from the typical gross appearance of renal cell carcinoma and so can usually be clearly separated. The tumours are well circumscribed and the cut surface has a uniform mahogany-brown colour without foci of haemorrhage or necrosis. Large oncocytomas commonly show a prominent stellate scar, which gives them a distinct gross appearance.

Microscopically, they are composed of large epithelial cells called oncocytes, which have abundant eosinophilic homogeneous or granular cytoplasm and uniform small nuclei. Electron microscopy shows these cells to be packed with abnormal mitochondria. Biochemical studies suggest a defect in mitochondrial ATP production with compensatory mitochondrial hyperplasia.

Mesenchymal tumours

1. Renomedullary interstitial cell tumour (medullary fibroma). These tumours cause virtually no symptoms and are noted as incidental findings at autopsy or nephrectomy for other reasons. They are small grey-white, well-circumscribed nodules, usually less than 1 cm in diameter, and located in the renal medulla.

Histologically, they are composed of small stellate or polygonal cells and bundles of delicate fibres in a loose myxoid matrix. Although also called fibroma, the tumour cells are not of fibroblast origin. At the periphery, renal medullary tubules are often entrapped in the matrix.

2. *Angiomyolipoma.* Angiolipomas are benign lesions characterized by the presence of mature adipose tissue, smooth muscle and thick-walled blood vessels. The true nature of these lesions is uncertain, but they are usually regarded as hamartomas. About 33% of patients with angiomyolipoma have tuberous sclerosis and more than 80% of tuberous sclerosis patients have angiomyolipoma.

Typically, the lesions are asymptomatic but may present with flank pain, mass, haematuria or a combination of these especially in patients with tuberous sclerosis. Grossly, the tumours are typically multifocal, bilateral and small in patients with tuberous sclerosis, and single, unilateral and large in those without. They are well circumscribed but not encapsulated and have varied appearances depending on the proportions of the constituent elements. In 25% of cases the tumours may be confused with malignancy because of extension outside the renal capsule.

3. *Juxtaglomerular cell tumour.* This is a rare, usually benign neoplasm of the juxtaglomerular cells of the kidney. Clinically, they occur mainly in young people, all of whom present with hypertension. Grossly, the tumours are small, usually less than 3 cm in diameter, well circumscribed and located in the cortex.

Embryonic tumours

1. Mesoblastic nephroma. This is a tumour that is usually found in the first 3 months of life and must be differentiated from nephroblastoma. The tumour varies in size from a small to very large mass that bulges from the kidney. It is hard in consistency and cut surface is white and whorled.

The tumour is composed of spindle cells and the margins are irregular with bands of tumour cells interdigitating with adjacent parenchyma. Mitoses are common but are normal as in other tissues of the rapidly growing infant.

The tumour is entirely benign. However, if tongues of tumour cells at the margins are left behind after surgical resection local recurrence is possible.

BLADDER CARCINOMA

Transitional cell carcinoma of the bladder (TCC) is the fourth most common cancer in men in the UK and USA. There are 64 000 new cases in the UK and USA each year. The high incidence of multiple tumours makes TCC the second most prevalent cancer in the UK. Seventy percent of patients present with superficial disease and two-thirds of these patients will develop recurrent tumour usually within 2–4 years. Since 1960 the incidence of bladder cancer has tripled, and recent statistics confirm that this trend is continuing. Cystoscopy remains the preferred and most accurate means for diagnosis of bladder carcinoma.

Risk factors

Bladder carcinoma is a disease of the elderly population. Males are more predominately affected than females (3:1) Carcinogens are causally associated with bladder TCC and include benzidine and β napthylamine. Occupations involving printing, dyeing, rubber and coal carry an increased risk together with laboratory and leather workers. There is also a strong association with smoking.

Presentation

Patients usually present over the age of 40 with painless haematuria. Other presentations include recurrent urinary tract infections, a sterile pyuria or lower urinary tract symptoms (LUTS) mostly irritative in nature (frequency, urgency, nocturia).

Investigations

1. Urine investigations. Urine cytology has a sensitivity of ~20% for superficial bladder cancer. Its use therefore is limited in the diagnosis and monitoring of the disease. Other urine tests such as the NMP22 (nuclear matrix protein) and BTA test (bladder tumour antigen) have increased sensitivity and specificity for detection of transitional cell carcinoma.

2. Imaging. IVP permits the imaging of the upper tracts as well as the bladder. Ureteric obstruction can occasionally be identified and tends to indicate muscle invasive disease. A bladder carcinoma is demonstrated as a filling defect. A postmicturition film often provides increased detail of the tumour extent. Ultrasound may also indicate the presence of a filling defect within the bladder. In many cases imaging may be negative.

3. Cystoscopy. Initial cystoscopic evaluation can be performed with a flexible instrument under local anaesthetic. It should be performed on all patients with a history of micro/macroscopic haematuria. The typical appearance of a superficial tumour is a luxuriant fronded structure arising from a flat surface. Red patches may indicate in situ disease.

Management

If a bladder tumour is detected a formal transurethral resection should be performed. The tumours are resected and the base is separately biopsied to assess the depth of disease. Careful bimanual examination is mandatory before and after surgery for staging purposes.

1. **Stage/Grade.** The histopathological criteria are extremely important for diagnosis but also for the subsequent management of the patient. The number and size of tumours at presentation may also affect the management.

- CIS *in situ* disease.
- pTa Papillary tumour confined to the mucosa and non-invasive (superficial).
- pT1 Subepithelial connective tissue invasion (locally invasive).
- pT2 Muscle invasion.
- pT3 Beyond muscle. Extravesical mass
- pT4a Involvement of prostate, uterus, vagina.
- T4b Pelvic side wall, abdominal wall.

2. Grades

1. Well differentiated.
2. Moderately differentiated.
3. Poorly differentiated.

Management of superficial and locally advanced disease

Superficial (pTa) and locally invasive (pT1) disease comprise 70% of all newly diagnosed bladder tumours. Follow-up is required not only to identify recurrent tumours but also detect disease progression. Within this group disease progression occurs in ~5% in 10 years. However, pT1G3 tumours have a progression rate to invasion/metastases of ~40% (29–63%) and with associated CIS this risk has been reported as high as 80%. These tumours require careful follow-up and should be treated more aggressively.

1. **Intravesical chemotherapy.** Intravesical chemotherapy is used to reduce the number of recurrent tumours and increase the recurrence-free interval. It is used for superficial and locally invasive disease only. This treatment has no impact on survival. It can be given within 6 hours of surgery as a single dose. It can also be given as a course of treatment for 'superficial' disease failing to respond to endoscopic resection and diathermy.

2. **Intravesical BCG.** Intravesical BCG is indicated for the treatment of CIS, pT1G3 tumours or failed intravesical chemotherapy. It has been developed from the virulent strain of *Mycobacterium bovis* and is a live attenuated organism. The exact mechanism of action is unclear, however it appears to offer superior results when compared with standard intravesical chemotherapy regimens and also reduces the incidence of disease progression.

3. **Other therapeutic options**

1. Laser. NdYag for tumour ablation.
2. Photodynamic therapy. The use of a tumour sensitizer (given intravenously) and laser light (given intravesically) for treatment of superficial disease.
3. Radiotherapy. Has a very limited application in superficial disease.
4. Cystectomy. May be required for uncontrollable superficial disease after failure of intravesical treatments.

Management of muscle invasive disease

Invasive TCC is far the commonest invasive bladder cancer (90–95%) comprising 30% of all TCC at presentation. Squamous cell carcinoma is common in schistosomiasis endemic areas. Adenocarcinoma represents only 1% of bladder cancers.

1. Investigation. Investigations should define the presence or absence of nodal and distant disease with a chest, abdominal and pelvic CT.

2. Treatments. The prognosis of patients with invasive bladder cancer is poor with most patients dying of metastatic disease. Patients with metastatic disease have a median survival of 6–12 months and those with regionally involved nodes have a median survival of 18 months. In order to improve survival patients with metastatic disease it is necessary to develop successful systemic treatment. Most patients are unfortunately too frail and elderly for multimodality treatments. The 5-year survival for muscle invasive bladder carcinoma ranges from 24–46%.

3. Cystectomy. Radical cystoprostatectomy (male) and radical anterior exenteration (female) appears to offer the best treatment option for invasive bladder carcinoma. Local recurrence rates are 10–20% but most patients will still die of distant metastases rather than local recurrence. Orthotopic bladder substitution (reconstructed bladder from small or large intestine sutured to the urethra) as the prime form of diversion after cystectomy continues to be favourable. It avoids a stoma but patients are likely to need to self-catheterize. Cystectomy with ileal diversion, however, continues as the most commonly performed operative technique.

4. Radiotherapy. Radiotherapy is a treatment option for invasive bladder carcinoma without metastatic spread. TCC are radiosensitive but SCC and adenocarcinoma less so. Although associated with a significant morbidity (dysuria, frequency and diarrhoea) it potentially cures 30% of patients. However, 50% of tumours will recur locally at 5 years. Nodal disease is not sensitive to radiotherapy and patients with CIS or squamous differentiation respond less well to radiotherapy.

5. Chemotherapy. TCC is chemosensitive with a response rate reported as high as 65% and complete response rates of 25%. Treatment with combination chemotherapy regimens (MVAC – Methotrexate, Vinblastine, Adriamycin and Cisplatin) appears to achieve remission in ~20% and a small but significant survival advantage has been demonstrated in small studies.

Further reading

Oosterlinck *et al.* Guidelines on Bladder Carcinoma. The EAU working group on Oncological Urology. *European Urology*, 2002; **41**: 105–112.

BLADDER TRAUMA

Bladder injuries occur as a result of blunt or penetrating trauma. A full bladder is more likely to become injured than an empty one.

Blunt trauma

Deceleration injuries usually produce both bladder trauma (perforation) and pelvic fractures. Approximately 10% of patients with pelvic fractures also have significant bladder injuries. The propensity of the bladder to sustain injury is related to its degree of distension at the time of trauma.

Penetrating trauma

Assault from a gunshot or stabbing typifies penetrating trauma. Often, concomitant abdominal and/or pelvic organ injuries are present.

Obstetric trauma

During prolonged labour or a difficult forceps delivery, persistent pressure from the fetal head against the mother's pubis can lead to bladder necrosis. Direct laceration of the urinary bladder is reported in 0.3% of women undergoing a caesarean delivery. Previous caesarean deliveries with resultant adhesions are a risk factor. Undue scarring may cause obliteration of normal tissue planes and facilitate an inadvertent extension of the incision into the bladder. Unrecognized bladder injuries may lead to vesico-uterine fistulas and other problems.

Gynaecologic trauma

Bladder injury may occur during a vaginal or abdominal hysterectomy. Blind dissection in the incorrect tissue plane between the base of the bladder and the cervical fascia results in bladder injury. Women with a history of pelvic radiation are at higher risk.

Urologic trauma

Perforation of the bladder during a bladder biopsy, cystolitholapaxy, transurethral resection of the prostate (TURP), or transurethral resection of a bladder tumour (TURBT) is not uncommon. Incidence of bladder perforation is reportedly as high as 36% following bladder biopsy.

Orthopaedic trauma

Orthopaedic pins commonly perforate the urinary bladder. Thermal injuries to the bladder wall may occur during the setting of cement substances used to seat arthroplasty prosthetics.

Idiopathic bladder trauma

Patients diagnosed with alcoholism and those individuals who chronically imbibe a large quantity of fluids are susceptible to this type of injury. Previous bladder surgery is a risk factor. In reported cases, all bladder ruptures were intraperitoneal. This type of injury may result from a combination of bladder overdistension and minor external trauma (e.g. a simple fall).

Pathophysiology

Bladder contusion is an incomplete or partial-thickness tear of the bladder mucosa. A segment of the bladder wall is bruised or contused, resulting in localized injury and haematoma. Contusion typically occurs in the following clinical situations:

- Patients presenting with gross haematuria after blunt trauma and normal imaging studies.
- Patients presenting with gross haematuria after extreme physical activity (i.e. long-distance running).

The bladder may appear normal or teardrop shaped on cystography. Bladder contusions are relatively benign, are the most common form of blunt bladder trauma, and are usually a diagnosis of exclusion. Bladder contusions are self-limiting and require no specific therapy, except for short-term bed rest until haematuria resolves. Persistent haematuria or unexplained lower abdominal pain requires further investigation.

Extraperitoneal bladder rupture

Traumatic extraperitoneal ruptures usually are associated with pelvic fractures (89–100%). Previously, the mechanism of injury was believed to be from a direct perforation by a bony fragment or a disruption of the pelvic girdle. It is now generally agreed that the pelvic fracture is likely coincidental and that the bladder rupture is most often due to a direct burst injury or the shearing force of the deforming pelvic ring.

Some cases may occur by a mechanism similar to intraperitoneal bladder rupture, which is a combination of trauma and bladder overdistension. The classic cystographic finding is contrast extravasation around the base of the bladder confined to the perivesical space; flame-shaped areas of contrast extravasation are noted adjacent to the bladder. The bladder may assume a teardrop shape from compression by a pelvic haematoma. Starburst, flame-shape and featherlike patterns are also described.

With a more complex injury, the contrast material extends to the thigh, penis, perineum or into the anterior abdominal wall. Extravasation will reach the scrotum when the superior fascia of the urogenital diaphragm or the urogenital diaphragm itself becomes disrupted.

If the inferior fascia of the urogenital diaphragm is violated, the contrast material will reach the thigh and penis (within the confines of the Colles fascia). Rarely, contrast may extravasate into the thigh through the obturator foramen or into the anterior abdominal wall. Sometimes, the contrast may extravasate through the inguinal canal and into the scrotum or labia majora.

Intraperitoneal bladder rupture

Classic intraperitoneal bladder ruptures are described as large horizontal tears in the dome of the bladder. The dome is the least supported area and the only portion of the adult bladder covered by peritoneum. This type of injury is common among patients diagnosed with alcoholism or those sustaining a seatbelt or steering wheel injury.

Since urine may continue to drain into the abdomen, intraperitoneal ruptures may go undiagnosed from days to weeks. Electrolyte abnormalities (e.g.

hyperkalaemia, hypernatraemia, uraemia, acidosis) may occur as urine is re-absorbed from the peritoneal cavity. Such patients may appear anuric, and the diagnosis is established when urinary ascites are recovered during paracentesis.

Intraperitoneal ruptures demonstrate contrast extravasation into the peritoneal cavity, often outlining loops of bowel, filling paracolic gutters, and pooling under the diaphragm. An intraperitoneal rupture is more common in children because of the relative intra-abdominal position of the bladder.

Clinical signs and diagnosis

Clinical signs of bladder injury are relatively non-specific; however, a triad of symptoms is often present (e.g. gross haematuria, suprapubic pain or tenderness, difficulty or inability to void).

Most patients with bladder rupture complain of suprapubic or abdominal pain, and many can still void; however, the ability to urinate does not exclude bladder injury or perforation. Haematuria invariably accompanies all bladder injuries. Gross haematuria is the hallmark of a bladder rupture. More than 98% of bladder ruptures are associated with gross haematuria, and 10% are associated with micro-scopic haematuria; conversely, 10% of patients with bladder ruptures have normal urinalyses.

An abdominal examination may reveal distension, guarding, or rebound tender-ness. Absent bowel sounds and signs of peritoneal irritation indicate a possible intraperitoneal bladder rupture.

In the setting of a motor vehicle accident or a crush injury, bilateral palpation of the bony pelvis may reveal abnormal motion indicating an open-book fracture or a disruption of the pelvic girdle.

If blood is present at the urethral meatus, suspect a urethral injury. Perform a ret-rograde urethrogram to assess the integrity of the urethra before attempting blindly to pass a urethral catheter. Blood at the urethral meatus is an absolute indication for retrograde urethrography. Approximately 10–20% of men with a posterior urethral injury have an associated bladder injury, therefore, do not place a urethral catheter in these patients. Passage of a urethral catheter may convert a partially disrupted urethra into a complete tear.

Place a urethral catheter only after urethral injuries are excluded. In the setting of a posterior urethral injury, insert a percutaneous suprapubic catheter.

Cystogram

Most patients have multiple injuries and require abdominal or pelvic CT scans as part of their trauma evaluation. This does not preclude obtaining a separate con-trast cystogram, since a CT scan of the pelvis using intravenous contrast alone is an unreliable study for bladder rupture.

A properly performed cystogram consists of an initial kidney–ureter–bladder (KUB), followed by anteroposterior (AP) and oblique views of the bladder filled with contrast, plus another AP film obtained after drainage. The following procedure is recommended:

- Obtain a plain radiograph.
- Place a urethral catheter in the bladder.
- Using a diluted contrast medium, slowly fill the bladder by gravity (approxi-mately 75 cm above the pelvis) to a volume of 300–400 cc. (Diluted contrast

media are usually 50% contrast and 50% sterile saline or water.) Use a contrast suitable for absorption.

- Obtain a single AP film of the pelvis and lower abdomen after the first 100 cc of contrast is instilled.
- If gross extravasation is noted, discontinue the procedure. If extravasation is absent, give the patient the remainder of the contrast.
- Obtain a KUB, followed by a post-drainage film of the pelvis.
- Obtain the post-drainage film after a complete drainage of the contrast. This is the most critical part of the study because it checks for extravasation that may be hidden by the distended bladder.
- If possible, obtain lateral and oblique films of the bladder. In children, obtain the estimated filling for the cystogram based on the following formula:

$$\text{Bladder capacity} = 60\,\text{cc} + (30\,\text{cc} \times \text{age in years})$$

If the patient is immediately taken to the operating room for an exploratory laparotomy and/or placement of a formal suprapubic cystostomy, the bladder is inspected at the time of surgery and the bladder injury is repaired. If surgery is delayed or an exploratory laparotomy is not contemplated, perform the cystogram via a percutaneous suprapubic tube (SPT) so that no bladder injury is overlooked.

Conservative therapy

Most extraperitoneal ruptures can be managed safely with simple catheter drainage (i.e. urethral or suprapubic). Leave the catheter in for 7–10 days, then obtain a cystogram. Approximately 85% of the time, the laceration is sealed and the catheter is removed for a voiding trial.

Virtually all extraperitoneal bladder injuries heal within 3 weeks. If the patient is taken to the operating room for associated injuries, extraperitoneal ruptures may be repaired concomitantly if the patient is stable.

Surgical therapy

1. *Intraperitoneal bladder rupture.* Most, if not all, intraperitoneal bladder ruptures require surgical exploration. These injuries do not heal with prolonged catheterization alone. Urine takes the path of least resistance and continues to leak into the abdominal cavity. This results in urinary ascites, abdominal distension and electrolyte disturbances.

Surgically explore all gunshot wounds to the lower abdomen. Because of the nature of associated visceral injuries, immediately take patients with high-velocity missile trauma to the operating room, where the bladder injuries can be repaired concomitantly with other visceral injuries.

Stab wounds to the suprapubic area involving the urinary bladder are managed selectively. Surgically repair obvious intraperitoneal injuries, and manage small extraperitoneal injuries expectantly with catheter drainage.

2. *Extraperitoneal extravasation.* Bladders with extensive extraperitoneal extravasation often are repaired surgically. Early surgical intervention decreases the length of hospitalization and potential complications, while promoting early recovery.

Further reading

Campbell MF, Retik AB, Darracott Vaughan E, Walsh PC. *Campbell's Urology*, 7th edn. WB Saunders Co, 1997.

Chapple C. Urethral injury. *BJU Int*, 2000; **86**: 318–326.

Corriere JN. Management of the ruptured bladder; seven years of experience with 111 cases. *Journal of Trauma*, 1986; 26: 830–833.

Korataitim MM. *Journal of Urology*, 1996; **156**: 1288–1291.

Webster GD. Prostatomembranous urethral injuries. *Journal of Urology*, 1983; **130**: 898–902.

CHRONIC END-STAGE RENAL FAILURE

Definition

Chronic renal failure (CRF) is a chronic deterioration in renal function resulting in a build-up of nitrogenous wastes in the plasma, together with a failure of the kidney to regulate extracellular fluid volume or composition. It is differentiated from acute renal failure mainly by its insidious onset and by its irreversible and progressive nature.

Aetiology

CRF may arise from a primary disorder of the kidney or may arise secondarily from the effects of a systemic disease on the kidney.

Renal causes can be further subdivided into glomerular and tubulointerstitial depending largely on the degree of proteinuria. >3.5 g/day suggests glomerular disease, <3.5 g/day suggests tubulointerstitial causes. Commoner forms of these types of disease, leading to CRF, are listed below.

1. Glomerular

- Focal segmental glomerulosclerosis.
- Membranous glomerulonephropathy.
- Membranoproliferative glomerulonephritis.
- Rapidly progressive glomerulonephritis.
- HIV-associated nephropathy.

2. Tubulointerstitial

- Autosomal dominant polycystic kidney disease (PKD).
- Juvenile PKD.
- Reflux nephropathy.
- Analgesic nephropathy.

In the western world, the commonest causes of CRF are diabetic nephropathy, hypertension and glomerulonephritis, accounting for almost 75% of cases.

Progression

It is well accepted that hypertension is one of the important factors in the progression of CRF. Importance of control of hypertension is well documented and has been shown to slow the rate of deterioration.

Clinical presentation

There are often no signs or symptoms of CRF as it is an insidious process. Symptoms tend not to occur until GFR has decreased to 30% of its original value. Symptoms at this stage are often related to the underlying disease process causing CRF, or are general in terms of malaise, lassitude, pruritis and confusion.

Investigation

- Urine
  - Infection
  - Protein (24 h)
  - Sodium
- Blood
  - Haemoglobin — Anaemia is the norm in CRF
  - Urea and creatinine — Raised
  - Bicarbonate — Chronic acidosis reduces the body's buffers
  - Potassium — Often normal until end stages
  - Phosphate — Hyperphosphataemia
  - Calcium — Hypocalcaemia common (secondary hyperparathyroidism)

Radiology

Contrast studies are to be avoided. Ultrasound scan will often add useful diagnostic information. Renal size and cortical thickness should always be assessed.

Biopsy

Renal biopsy may be diagnostic. Helpful in those with normal sized kidneys.

Management

In all cases the initial efforts should be to search for any reversible insults to renal function, as in ARF. Assuming no reversible factors are identified, initial management is conservative. Conservative management can be grouped into three areas:

1. Prevent additional insults to renal function.
2. Treat complications of CRF.
3. Attempt to slow progression.

In practical terms this means giving careful attention to management of any underlying disease process, such as diabetes, treating and controlling hypertension rigorously, correcting anaemia and restricting dietary intake of nitrogen, potassium and sodium. Avoiding nephrotoxic drugs such as tetracyclines, nitrofurantoin, aminoglycosides, amiloride, spironolactone and NSAIDs.

Renal replacement

Only in those where conservative management has failed should renal replacement be considered and dialysis commenced.

Indications for dialysis

All indications are relative and are assessed on an individual patient basis.

- Hyperkalaemia >6 mmol/l and uncontrolled by other means.
- Urea >20 mmol/l.
- Creatinine >500 mmol/l.
- Bicarbonate <12 mmol/l.
- Symptoms or signs of uraemia.

 The ideal form of renal replacement is renal transplantation. Sadly, there are not enough donor organs and therefore other forms of renal replacement need to be instituted in the short and often the long term.

Chronic ambulatory peritoneal dialysis

The peritoneum here provides the dialysis 'membrane'. Access to the peritoneal cavity is by a soft Tenckoff catheter. Sterile dialysate solution is infused into the peritoneal cavity and drained off at prescribed intervals through the day.

1. Pros

- Convenience – allows for free mobility and can be performed at home.
- Cost.
- Ease of establishing peritoneal access.

2. Cons

1. Peritonitis. This is a common complication of CAPD but usually follows a benign course and can be managed successfully by antibiotics and conservative measures. Common organisms responsible are *S. epidermidis* and *S. aureus*.
2. Protein energy malnutrition and other metabolic complications.

Haemodialysis

Access is usually accomplished by surgical creation of an arteriovenous fistula in the upper limb. Blood is pumped across a cupraphane or cellulose acetate membrane to remove body solutes and excess fluid. Normal dialysis regimens are for 4 h a day, 3 days a week

1. Pros

- Effective.
- More versatile than CAPD.

2. Cons

- Expense.
- Rarely available at home.
- Requires anticoagulation.

Complications of CRF and dialysis

- Pericarditis and pericardial effusion.
- Infection.
- Hypotension.
- Myocardial ischaemia.
- Dialysis dysequilibrium syndrome – weakness, dizziness, headache and possible mental state changes.

Unfortunately, despite all the advances in dialysis techniques the mortality figures for CRF remain about 20% and there still remains an acute shortage of donor kidneys for transplantation.

CHRONIC PYELONEPHRITIS

Definition

The term 'chronic pyelonephritis' refers to renal injury caused by either recurrent or persistent infection. It is commonly associated with anatomical anomalies in the affected kidney. These may include:

- Urinary tract obstruction.
- Renal dysplasia.
- Struvite calculi.
- Vesico ureteric reflux.

Pathophysiology

Chronic pyelonephritis is associated with progressive renal scarring which can ultimately lead to end-stage renal disease. The mechanism for this is thought to be intra-renal reflux of infected urine inducing renal injury and then healing by scar formation. This in turn can lead to some of the clinical sequelae of:

- Proteinuria.
- Hypertension.
- Focal glomerulosclerosis.
- End-stage renal disease.

Chronic pyelonephritis is more common in females than males and can occur either in childhood or adulthood.

Clinical presentation

Patients with chronic pyelonephritis may complain of the following:

- Fever.
- Lethargy.
- Nausea and vomiting.
- Flank pain.
- Dysuria.
- Usually pain is the predominant feature.

Examination

- Signs of fever.
- Loin tenderness.
- Hypertension.
- Failure to thrive in children.

Investigation

1. Urine

- Pus cells.
- Bacteria: *E. coli* and *Proteus* are the most common.
- Proteinuria.

Negative urine culture does, however, not exclude the diagnosis.

2. Blood tests. The following may be present:

- Raised white cell count.
- Elevated serum urea and creatinine.

3. Imaging

- Intravenous urogram can be diagnostic showing the typical features of chronic pyelonephritis, calyceal dilatation with calyceal blunting and cortical scarring. Ureteric dilatation may be visible along with a reduction in renal size.
- Ultrasound may show reduced renal size and renal scarring.
- Radioisotope scanning with DMSA (technetium dimercaptosuccinic acid) is the most sensitive method for detecting renal scarring.
- Micturating cystogram may show evidence of vesicoureteric reflux, but involves a relatively high dose of radiation to the pelvis and should not be regarded as a routine investigation.

Management

Any underlying condition such as stones, obstruction or vesico ureteric reflux should be treated.

1. Conservative. Medical therapy with antibiotics such as amoxycillin, trimethoprim or nitrofurantoin may be sufficient to control symptoms. These antibiotics should however be continued long term at low dose (i.e. one tablet at night).

Such antibiotic therapy should be continued until puberty or until the resolution of reflux in those children presenting with the disease.

2. Surgical intervention. This should be restricted to those cases where medical therapy has failed to control infections or symptoms.

Essentially there are only two forms of surgical intervention:

1. Surgery to correct an underlying abnormality, such as vesicoureteric reflux.
2. Nephrectomy to give symptomatic relief from a chronically scarred painful kidney.

Xanthogranulomatous pyelonephritis (XPN)

This is a rare, severe subset of chronic pyelonephritis occurring in about 8%. It is a severe chronic renal infection typically resulting in diffuse renal destruction. Most cases tend to be unilateral and result in a non-functioning enlarged kidney associated often with obstructive uropathy secondary to nephrolithiasis. The peak incidence is in the age range 50–70 and women are three times more commonly affected than men. 15% of patients are diabetic. The most common organism involved is *Proteus* with *E. coli* a close second.

Part of its importance is that it is a great imitator of a renal tumour and CT scan is often needed to distinguish them. XPN usually appears as a renal mass with the renal pelvis surrounding a central area of calcification but with no dilatation of the renal pelvis.

Management

Nephrectomy is often required to control symptoms of pain and recurrent infection. This procedure is often technically extremely challenging with granulomatous tissue extending to the great vessels and even to the diaphragm. It is not a procedure to be undertaken lightly.

DETRUSOR INSTABILITY

The functions of the bladder and lower urinary tract are storage and timely expulsion of urine, plus maintenance of a barrier between urine and plasma. The bladder is capable of accomplishing its storage function by accepting volumes of urine with little or no change in intravesical pressures. Continence is maintained by the sphincters of the bladder neck (internal sphincter) and the striated muscle of the urethral sphincter (external sphincter). Micturition is a finely tuned event coordinated by the opening of the sphincters and detrusor muscle contraction.

According to the International Continence Society (ICS) the 'unstable detrusor' is one that is shown objectively to contract, spontaneously or on provocation, during the bladder filling phase while the patient is attempting to inhibit micturition.

The generic term for involuntary detrusor contractions is detrusor overactivity. When involuntary detrusor contractions are caused by neurological pathology, the condition is called detrusor hyperreflexia. In the absence of a neurological pathology the condition is termed detrusor instability.

Symptoms typical of detrusor instability are:

- Frequency
  Nocturia.
  Urgency.
  Urge incontinence.
  Nocturnal enuresis.

Once urinary incontinence is reported, an initial evaluation should focus on the severity of urinary leakage and the patient's goals for resolution of the problem. The urinary diary is a mainstay of incontinence evaluation. This simple instrument allows the patient to record voided volumes, leakage episodes (and amounts), and volume of fluid intake. Although a 3- to 5-day diary is optimal, a single typical 24-h period is more appropriate.

The possible aetiology of the detrusor instability

Condition	Examples
Bladder outlet obstruction	BPH, urethral stricture
Neurological disease	Multiple sclerosis, stroke, spinal cord injury, Parkinsonism, diabetes
Irradiation and chemical cystitis	Following irradiation of pelvic tumours of prostate, rectum and cervix
Bladder neoplasm and carcinoma in situ	
Anatomic defects	Urethral hypermobility and deficiency cystocele, uterine prolapse, pregnancy
Idiopathic	
Psychogenic	
Neurotransmitter imbalance	Depression, psychiatric patients on treatment

Investigations

1. MSSU. Cystoscopy is indicated in the presence of abnormal urine microscopy/ culture where it is important to exclude intravesical pathology such as bladder tumour or stone.

Disorders of detrusor motor function can be demonstrated with the use of filling and voiding cystometry (urodynamics). It also gives us the opportunity to diagnose bladder outlet obstruction.

Treatment of detrusor instability

1. Pharmacological

   - Oral   Tolderodine (anticholinergic)
     Oxybutynin (anticholinergic)
     Tricyclic antidepressants

   - Intravesical   Capsaicin
     Resiniferatoxin
     Oxybutynin

2. Electrical stimulation   Sacral nerve stimulation

3. Surgery   Urethrolysis
    Augmentation cystoplasty

4. Behaviour modification

Anticholinergics are competitive inhibitors of acetylcholine that block its muscarinic effects. All of the active drugs must be given in an adequate dosage to ensure a physiological effect. In practice, the dosage may be increased every 3–5 days until the patient improves clinically or until untoward side-effects, such as dry mouth, blurred vision or supraventricular tachycardia. Anticholinergics are contraindicated in patients with untreated closed angle glaucoma.

Intravesical agents have been tried as alternatives to oral medication. This offers high drug concentrations at the detrusor muscle level and also avoids systemic side-effects.

Surgery is only indicated occasionally in patients with refractory detrusor instability. Therapies such as denervation, augmentation cystoplasty, myomectomy, urinary diversion and rhizotomy are used in exceptional circumstances. Almost all surgical therapies are designed, in one way or another, to circumvent the problems. None of the procedures abolish detrusor instability and restore normal micturition. When detrusor instability is abolished by surgical intervention, detrusor contractility is also adversely altered, and subsequent bladder emptying relies on abdominal straining or self-intermittent catheterization.

Sacral nerve stimulation (SNS) is somatic afferent inhibition of sensory processing in the spinal cord. The electrodes for SNS are usually placed through the S3 sacral foramen. These are then attached to a TENS unit-like pulse generator and stimulated appropriately. Studies have demonstrated significant improvement in the reduction of urge incontinence episodes and pads used per day over a 6-month period.

Behaviour modification is an effective way of treatment as it teaches the patient to regain control of the bladder and sphincter. The principles are quite simple. For example the patient maintains a weekly voiding diary. Fluid restriction is recommended to decrease output. In addition patients are taught muscle contracting techniques such as Kegel exercises, which are used to abort involuntary detrusor contractions.

Further reading

Kurth H. Control of bladder function: the overactive bladder. *BJU Int*, 1999; **83(2)**.

DIATHERMY

Diathermy is integral to the practice of urology. It relies on the safe and effective conversion of mains alternating current (50 Hz) to the radiofrequency range (300–3000 Hz) and application of this energy to tissues. The high frequency energy heats tissues and, dependent on its waveform, it will either cut or coagulate tissue. The energy can be applied to the tissues in two forms: monopolar and bipolar. Generators are of two types, isolated and earthed, though the former is safest and most frequently used.

Cutting (125–250 W)

The wave form applied to the tissues is a pure sine wave. This will essentially vaporize tissue in direct contact with the electrode but will not spread tangentially and coagulate tissue.

Coagulation (40–75 W)

The waveform is interrupted and usually of a higher peak energy. This does not cause vaporization but dries and seals tissue. Smooth muscle in vessel walls.

Blended current

This waveform of ac applied to the tissue is a constant sine wave but the amplitude (i.e., energy applied) is variable similar to coagulation; however it never returns to zero. It both cuts and coagulates.

Monopolar

The energy generated by the diathermy machine is applied to tissues with a relatively fine instrument (e.g. forceps) – the so-called 'active electrode' – and causes heating or vaporization of these tissues. This energy must then find its way to earth and to allow this a passive electrode is sited. This is usually an aluminium pad with or without adhesive applied to the patient's leg. The pad is of a much larger area than the active electrode to prevent heating and burning of tissue.

Bipolar

Currently, bipolar diathermy is only available to coagulate and can be applied through forceps or scissors. The active and passive electrodes are combined in the delivery system and will not work if the metal of the forceps are in contact with each other.

Diathermy safety

1. Burns

- If the passive electrode is non-adhesive and contact is poor or wet a large burn may occur.
- Direct contact between the operating table and plate should be avoided.
- If an earthed machine is used and the passive plate is faulty, current will earth via the ECG monitor pads.

2. Explosions

- Avoid using alcohol as skin prep especially in areas where pooling may occur (skin creases, umbilicus).
- Do not diathermy vigorously in the gas bubble at the time of cystoscopy explosion and bladder rupture has been reported.

Fault finding

1. Machine alarming

- Check the passive electrode (connection, application and integrity).
- Check the passive electrode cable (integrity and connection).
- Check the active electrode (cable and connection).

2. Poor or non-function

- Check the passive electrode (cable, connection and integrity).
- Check the active electrode (cable, connection, clean).
- Check the foot or finger switch.
- Check the machine (turned on).
- At cystoscopy check the irrigant (should not be saline).

Further reading

Kramolowsky KV, Tucker RD. The urological applications of electrosurgery. *Journal of Urology*, 1991; **146**: 669–674.

Perlmutter *et al*. Advances in electrosurgical techniques. *Current Opinion in Urology*, 1997; **7**: 21–24.

EPIDIDYMO-ORCHITIS

In men younger than 35 years of age epididymo-orchitis is most often caused by sexually transmitted pathogens such as *Chlamydia trachomatis* and *Neisseria gonorrhoeae*. In men older than 35 years of age epididymo-orchitis is most often caused by non-sexually transmitted Gram-negative enteric organisms causing urinary tract infections.

Gram-negative enteric organisms are more commonly the cause of epididymo-orchitis if recent instrumentation or catheterization has occurred. Anatomical abnormalities of the urinary tract are common in the group infected with Gram-negative enteric organisms and further investigation of the urinary tract should be considered in all such patients, but especially in those older than 50 years.

Epididymo-orchitis has been described in 12–19% of men with Behçet's disease. This is non-infective and thought to be part of the disease process. Epididymo-orchitis has also been reported as an adverse effect of amiodarone treatment.

Presentation

Patients with epididymo-orchitis usually present with unilateral testicular pain. In sexually transmitted epididymo-orchitis there may be symptoms of a urethritis or a urethral discharge; however, the urethritis is often asymptomatic. Torsion of the spermatic cord (testicular torsion) is the main differential diagnosis. This is a surgical emergency. Torsion should be considered in all patients and should be excluded first as testicular salvage becomes decreasingly likely with time.

Clinical signs

There may be tenderness to palpation on the affected side and palpable swelling of the epididymis. They may also be:

- Urethral discharge.
- Hydrocele.
- Erythema and/or oedema of the scrotum on the affected side.
- Pyrexia.

Diagnosis

Microscopy and culture of mid-stream urine for bacteria should be performed. If the condition is suspected to be sexually transmitted then a nucleic acid amplification test or antigen detection test for *C. trachomatis* of first void urine or urethral swab should be performed. A nucleic acid test amplification test is preferable as it is much more sensitive.

Colour Doppler ultrasound is useful to help differentiate between epididymo-orchitis and torsion of the spermatic cord.

Management

Bed rest, scrotal elevation and support, and analgesics are recommended. Non-steroidal anti-inflammatory drugs may be helpful. Patients should be advised to avoid unprotected sexual intercourse until they and their partner(s) have completed treatment and follow-up.

Further investigation

All patients with sexually transmitted epididymo-orchitis should be screened for other sexually transmitted infections.

Treatment

Empirical therapy should be given to all patients with epididymo-orchitis before culture results are available. The antibiotic regimen chosen should be determined in light of the immediate tests as well as age, sexual history, any recent instrumentation or catheterization, and any known urinary tract abnormalities in the patient.

- Ciprofloxacin 500 mg by mouth single dose.

plus

- Doxycycline 100 mg by mouth twice daily for 10–14 days.

Sexual partners

If the epididymo-orchitis is caused by, or likely to be caused by, a sexually transmitted pathogen such as *N. gonorrhoeae* or *C. trachomatis* then sexual contacts must be evaluated.

Patients may require admission to hospital. If the symptoms fail to settle then an ultrasound scan of the testes is important. This may help to exclude testicular ischaemia/infarction, abscess formation and testicular or epididymal tumour.

Mumps epididymo-orchitis, tuberculous epididymitis and fungal epididymitis also need to be considered with failed conventional antibiotic treatment.

EPISPADIAS AND BLADDER EXSTROPHY COMPLEX

Classification

1. Isolated epispadias.
2. Classical bladder exstrophy.
3. Cloacal exstrophy.

Demography

This occurs in 1/50 000 live births, the majority being classic exstrophy, with cloacal exstrophy representing 10%. Male infants are affected 3–4 times more frequently. As yet no method of inheritance or aetiological factors have been identified.

Embryology

In early embryonic life the cloaca forms from the hindgut distal to the allantois. This area is then further subdivided into the urogenital sinus and rectum by caudal growth of the urorectal septum and this is usually complete by 7 weeks. By this stage of development mesenchyme anterior to the urogenital sinus has condensed to form the genital tubercule. The lower anterior abdominal wall develops between the genital tubercle and the umbilicus.

Clinical features

1. Epispadias. The urethral meatus opens on the dorsal aspect of the penis and is classified as glanular, penile and penopubic. The glans is bifid and a groove extends from the glans to the meatus. If the meatus is sited in the penile or penopubic area the rhabdosphincter is deficient and the child is incontinent. The penis is short, broad and chordee is present. This defect is probably due to the genital tubercle developing in relatively caudal position.

2. Classical exstrophy. The anterior bladder wall is deficient and the umbilicus relatively low. The genitalia are epispadiac and the pubic bones widely separated. In this case the genital tubercle has developed in a caudal position and in addition the anterior abdominal wall has failed to develop.

3. Cloacal exstrophy. This is a severe defect and is associated with multiple gastrointestinal abnormalities along with bifid genitalia and bladder. The rectum and bladder both empty onto the anterior abdominal wall and the colon is often prolapsed. The pubic symphysis is again widely separated.

Management

These defects should be managed in a specialist unit. Initially the umbilicus should be ligated with silk to prevent erosion of the exposed bladder. The defect should then be covered with a plastic membrane to prevent desiccation. The principles of repair are:

1. Bladder closure.
2. Bladder neck reconstruction.
3. Ureteric reimplantation.
4. Penile reconstruction/urethroplasty.

Usually the bladder is closed in the early neonatal period – this results in a small capacity bladder and ureteric reflux is the rule. To achieve bladder closure the pubic bones are sutured together and may require osteotomy to allow closure. The penis and urethra (epispadias repair) are usually reconstructed in the first year of life. Bladder neck reconstruction to allow continence is performed before the child goes to school and the ureters are reimplanted and the bladder augmented as necessary. Alternatively the whole repair can be performed in one stage.

Further reading

Baker LA, Gearhart JP. The staged approach to bladder exstrophy closure and the role of osteotomies. *World Journal of Urology*, 1998; **16**: 205–211.
www.pediatrics.org

ERECTILE DYSFUNCTION

Erectile dysfunction is the persistent inability to obtain or maintain a penile erection adequate for coitus. It affects approximately one in seven men with increasing incidence with age.

Pathogenesis

Erectile dysfunction occurs as a result of either psychological or organic factors. Organic factors such as endocrine, vasculogenic and neurological are often associated with psychological factors.

The erectile mechanism

Blood flow into the erectile tissue (corpora) is controlled by smooth muscle tone. In the flaccid state a high peripheral resistance caused by smooth muscle contraction allow minimal blood to enter the erectile tissue. Relaxation by the release of neurotransmitters allows arterial vasodilatation and expansion of the erectile tissue. This expansion causes the penis to lengthen and blood is trapped within the penis as the veins surrounding the erectile tissue are compressed.

Causes of organic erectile dysfunction

Local	Systemic
Arterial – Arteriosclerosis	**Drugs** (β-blockers; spironolactone; methyldopa)
Neurological – CNS trauma	**Endocrine** – Diabetes mellitus
Anatomical ⟨ Post-surgical / Venous leak	**Infection** – Prostatitis
	Renal failure
	Advanced prostate cancer

History and investigations

A medical and sexual history are important in order to try and differentiate organic from psychological causes. Patients can sometimes interpret impotence erroneously as lack of libido or premature ejaculation.

A full examination including genitalia and peripheral pulses. A rectal examination is mandatory. A routine haematological and biochemical analysis will help to exclude many of the systemic causes. More specialized tests such as FSH/LH; testosterone; prolactin may also be required for the evaluation of endocrine function in the assessment of erectile dysfunction.

Specialized investigations

The use of arterial colour duplex ultrasonography with cavernosometry and cavernosography for assessment of venous leakage are only performed in specialized centres and have limited use in the routine decision-making for patient treatment.

Treatments

Careful consideration to treatment is given after consultation with the patient and his partner. Treatments continue to change with the introduction of effective oral preparations. Therapy may include oral medication, mechanical aids or surgery and psychotherapy.

1. Oral medication. The mainstay of this treatment is to facilitate smooth muscle relaxation.

- Sildenafil (Viagra doses of 50–100 mg used 2–3 times per week – contraindicated with nitrates).

This medication works as a potent inhibitor of cyclic guanosine monophosphate (GMP), specific type 5, which is the enzyme responsible for the breakdown of cyclic GMP in the corpora. This results in a build-up of cyclic GMP which will cause smooth muscle relaxation and arteriole expansion. The main side effects are flushing, headache and dyspepsia. A response of ~70% has been seen in a dose escalation study for successful coitus as compared with 22% for placebo. Patients with diabetes have an improved erection response of ~50% when using 50 mg.

- Trazadone (100–200 mg doses on demand).

This medication is a centrally acting serotoninergic agonist. It appears to work in approximately 60% of patients and may have more promising results in patients with psychogenic erectile dysfunction.

- Phentolamine mesylate (40–80 mg on demand).

There is an increased adrenergic tone especially in older men stimulated through pre- and post-synaptic junctional pathways in corporal smooth muscle and α-adrenergic stimulation has a negative effect on erectile function. The use of α_1- and α_2-adrenergic receptor blockade looks promising but is still in the development stage.

2. Topical and transurethral therapy. The use of topical preparations including patches have not been shown to have good results. One of the main problems is diffusion of the drug across penile skin. A viable alternative is intra-urethral treatment.

- Trans-urethral alprostadil MUSE (doses of 250–1000 µg).

This form of treatment comes as a pellet which is placed after voiding in the distal urethra with a supplied applicator. A condom is recommended and a constriction ring may be placed at the base of the penis to improve the erection. Alprostadil is a synthetic form of prostaglandin-E1 and smooth muscle relaxation is mediated through cyclic AMP. Studies have shown response rates sufficient for intercourse to vary between 30–60%.

3. Intra-cavernosal drugs. This form of treatment is rapidly becoming second-line treatment as a result of the introduction of oral medications. Most of the drugs are extremely effective (>90%) and safe for long-term treatment. The drug is administered by injection directly into the corpora. Patients are taught self-injection following a dose escalation in the clinic to prevent the potential problems of priapism.

- Alprostadil (doses of 2.5–40 µg).

Alprostadil not only has an effect through the cyclic AMP pathway to facilitate smooth muscle relaxation but also adrenergic vasoconstrictor tone.

- Paperverine.

This drug is a non-selective phosphodiesterase inhibitor and causes smooth muscle relaxation by increasing the levels of cyclic GMP in the tissues. It has a high incidence of priapism and can cause fibrosis at the site of injection. Because of the acidity of the solution there is an increased incidence of pain at the injection site.

In conclusion there are numbers of pharmaceutical options which differ in their mode of action. Combination of therapies utilizing different biochemical pathways are also used for those patients refractory to single therapy.

4. Mechanical aids. These treatments are suitable for patients in which pharmaceutical agents are contraindicated or do not work. They generally consist of a cylinder into which the penis is placed and a vacuum created by a manual or electric pump. This has the effect of drawing blood into the corpora and venous leakage is prevented by the use of a constriction ring at the base of the penis. The problems are that only the part of the penis visible becomes erect and will also result in a 'cold' erect penis.

5. Surgery. Surgery to improve arterial inflow and prevent venous leakage has limited success but is useful for carefully selected cases performed in highly specialized units. A number of rigid and inflatable penile prostheses are also available.

Further reading

Wespes E *et al.* Guidelines on erectile dysfunction. *Eur Urol,* 2002; **41**: 1–5.

EXTRACORPOREAL SHOCK WAVE LITHOTRIPSY (ESWL)

History

Sound waves were first used to fragment calculi in Russia in the 1950s. The concept was rediscovered by Dornier in subsequent years. The first lithotripsy applied to humans using the Dornier HM1 in 1980. This was refined leading to the HM2 and 3 models and subsequently numerous manufacturers have joined the market. The results were initially published in 1982 by Chaussy.

Physics

Shock waves focused at a point produce a rapid increase in pressure with subsequent steep fall to below normal pressure at the focal point. There is then recovery to the baseline normal pressure at a relatively slower rate. This results in erosion at the entry and exit portions of the calculus due to cavitation and shearing forces are created within the stone which cause it to shatter. A portion of the shock wave is reflected backwards resulting in further shearing forces and shattering.

Generation of shock wave

A reliable electric current is necessary for shock wave generation. This is either applied between two electrodes with a resultant explosive spark (spark gap, super-sonic emission) across a ceramic plate (piezoelectric, finite amplitude emission) or to produce electromagnetic motion in a sheet of metal (finite amplitude emission). All three devices require focusing mechanisms to concentrate shock waves on the calculus.

Indications

1. Renal pelvic calculus less than 2 cm.
2. Calyceal calculus less than 1.5 cm.
3. Upper ureteric calculus (*in situ*) less than 1 cm.
4. Lower ureteric calculus.
5. Combined therapy ('sandwich') with percutaneous nephrolithotomy (PCNL) for Staghorn calculus.

Contra-indications

1. *Absolute contra-indications*

- Pregnancy.
- Uncorrectable coagulopathy.

2. *Relative contra-indications*

- Sepsis.
- Anti-coagulant therapy (aspirin, warfarin).
- Severe obesity.
- Cardiac pacemaker (unless cardiologist in attendance).
- Urinary tract obstruction.

Patient selection

A recent IVU or retrograde pyelo-ureterogram is mandatory to delineate the upper tract anatomy and accurately localize the calculus. Outcome in dilated systems and for calculi within dependent calyces with long narrow infundibulae or within calyceal diverticulae is less favourable.

Provision of lithotripsy

1. Within a tertiary referral stone centre, treatment is usually supervised by a senior member of the medical staff.
2. Mobile lithotripsy units, treatment is usually supervised by a radiographer or nurse with training in the field with any medical input provided by a member of the medical staff within the hospital. Occasionally if this mobile unit is connected to a tertiary referral centre a medical officer may accompany the unit.

Procedure of lithotripsy

1. KUB on day of treatment.
2. Exclude/treat infection (dipstix for nitrates/white cells).
3. Informed consent.
4. Pre-medication – analgesia (for example Diclofenac sodium 100 mg per rectum) with an anti-emetic or antibiotic as needed.
5. Positioning: prone for lower ureteral calculi, supine for renal or upper ureteric calculi, lateral rotation to remove bony obstructions from the field.
6. Localization of calculus – ultrasound or fluoroscopic methods. May require intravenous or retrogradely administered contrast.
7. Monitoring, mandatory ECG as cardiac dysrhythmia may occur, blood pressure/pulse/SaO_2 if opiate analgesia used. In adults patient-controlled analgesia and also general anaesthesia are sometimes necessary; for young children general anaesthesia is more acceptable to patient, parent and doctor.

Post-lithotripsy

1. Advise profuse oral fluids and rapid mobilization.
2. Provide adequate analgesia and define a point of contact should there be any significant problems (usually the on-call urology Senior House Officer).
3. Review appointments at out-patients between 2–6 weeks dependent on local protocols.
4. Ask patient to strain the urine and collect any calculus debris for later metabolic analysis.

Adverse events post-lithotripsy

1. Renal

- Haematuria, essentially normal after lithotripsy.
- Peri-renal haematoma (less than 1% of cases) presents with severe loin pain not responding to simple analgesics. Investigate as per blunt renal trauma.
- Renal rupture, very rare and may require open renal exploration.
- Hypertension; as yet no definitive link has been proven.

2. *Ureteric complications – Steinstrasse.* Obstruction of the ureteric lumen by impacted fragments. If asymptomatic regular radiographic surveillance will suffice. Sepsis requires emergency intervention with percutaneous nephrostomy and antibiotics. This decompresses the ureter and allows ureteric contraction and may allow expulsion of the stones. If there is no change in the Steinstrasse ureteroscopic dis-impaction of the fragments can be considered. Usually there is one large fragment at the head of the Steinstrasse which when removed allows free drainage.

3. *Surrounding tissues*

- Cutaneous bruising.
- Pancreatitis (especially on the left side and is very rare).

Further reading

Chow GK *et al.* Extracorporeal lithotripsy – update on technology. *Urology Clinics of North America*, 2000; **27**: 315–322.

GENITOURINARY TUBERCULOSIS (TB)

TB can affect any organ in the urinary tract and is characterized by a chronic granulomatous inflammation. Infection is invariably via the haematogenous route from the lungs. The kidney is usually the site of initial infection and the other organs are infected by shedding of organisms into the urine. The epididymis and testicle are affected by direct spread along the vas. Its peak incidence is between 20–40 years and shows a slight male preponderance.

Symptoms

- Renal disease – usually asymptomatic.
- Ureteric disease – loin pain if kidney functioning.
- Bladder – Frequency, urgency, bladder pain, haematuria.
- Genital – painless epididymal swelling or discharging scrotal sinus.

Investigations

1. Bacteriological

MSSU
- Classical feature is sterile pyuria.
- 20% will be associated with bacturia.

Early morning urine (EMU)
- The first voided sample of urine is collected.
- Microscopy performed after staining with Ziehl-Neelsen.

Prostate secretions
- Prostate massage may be performed if the gland is indurated.

2. Radiology

Plain abdominal film
- Calcification of the renal parenchyma.
- Prostate/seminal vesicle calcification.

Chest X-ray
- Calcification of lung may indicate the primary infection.

Intravenous urogram
- Calcification of the renal parenchyma.
- Ulcerated calyces.
- Calyceal dilatation due to infundibular stenosis.
- Ureteric stricture.
- Non-functioning kidney with contralateral hypertrophy.

Treatment

1. Medical

- Combination medical therapy.

  Isoniazid ⎫
  Rifampicin ⎪
  Etambutol ⎬ combination of three agents
  Streptomycin ⎪
  Pyrazinamide ⎭

- A 6-month course is recommended.
- Further treatment if cultures remain positive.

2. Surgical

- Nephrectomy
  - Non-function.
  - Persistent culture.
  - After 2 months medical therapy.

- Cystoplasty
  - Severe bladder contracture.
  - Augmentation.
  - Substitution (partial cystectomy).

- Orchidectomy
  - Failed medical therapy.

Follow-up

- Urine culture on a 6-monthly basis for 10 years.
- Active surveillance of renal units to prevent hydronephrosis/renal loss.

Further reading

Weiss SG *et al.* Genitourinary tuberculosis. *Urology*, 1998; **51**: 1033–1034.

HYPOSPADIAS

Demography

This remains commonest genital abnormality affecting approximately 1 in 300 boys. There is an increased risk of this defect in siblings (14%) and offspring (8%) of a hypospadiac patient. No distinct method of inheritance has as yet been identified. Hypospadias is associated with increased incidence of testicular maldescent (9–30%) and around 1 in 10 have an associated inguinal hernia.

Embryology

At 5 weeks of gestation the fetal genitalia are ambiguous and under the influence of androgens (probably dihydrotestosterone (DHT)). The genitalia develop along male lines. The urethra forms from the flat urethral plate and should be complete and tubularized by around 15 weeks of gestation. The foreskin also develops again probably under the influence of DHT and is complete by around 25 weeks.

Aetiology

The exact aetiology of hypospadias is unknown but the presence of hypospadiac genitalia in boys with 5α reductase deficiency implies that DHT is involved. Recent publications have implied maternal vegetarianism, iron supplementation and influenza infection in pregnancy are linked with this abnormality. Maternal treatment with stilboestrol or oestrogens has also been implicated.

Clinical features

The classical hypospadias complex consists of:

- Hooded foreskin (deficient ventrally).
- Chordee (ventral penile angulation).
- Abnormally sited ventral urethral meatus.

Classification

Hypospadias is classified dependent on the position of the meatus:

- Glanular ⎫
- Coronal ⎬ 50%
- Penile   20%
- Penoscrotal ⎫
- Perineal   ⎬ 30%

Investigations

If associated with impalpable testes the child requires investigation to ascertain the genetic sex and exclude salt wasting metabolic congenital adrenal hyperplasia. If the infant has non-urinary tract malformations it is wise to assess the kidneys with ultrasound.

Management

The surgical repair of glandular and coronal hypospadias is essentially cosmetic and can be delayed into adulthood. More proximal defects require surgery to allow the boy to void in the standing position and allow him to direct the stream of urine. These procedures are usually performed before the stage of genital awareness (<2 years). The essential steps of repair are:

- Glanuloplasty (recontructing a cosmetically acceptable glans).
- Orthoplasty (correction of chordee).
- Urethroplasty (formation of urethra and an acceptable meatus).
- Adequate skin cover/cosmesis.

Well over 100 techniques described to repair hypospadias, in one or two stages. All bar simple meatal advancement or very distal defects require the urine to be diverted post-operatively to protect the suture line – usually within infant feeding tube sutured in place and passed through a double nappy. The essentials of successful repair are to use well-vascularized tissue, avoidance of tension at suture lines, a waterproofing layer and avoidance of infection. The urethroplasty is commonly performed using the inner layer of the prepuce, penile skin or buccal mucosa. Historically bladder mucosa has been used but harvesting is difficult. Buccal mucosa is rapidly becoming the tissue of choice for urethroplasty as it is easy to harvest, in plentiful supply, is designed to be wet and has the added advantage of conservation of preputial skin. The main problems associated with repair are fistula formation (15–30%), urethral/meatal stricture, urethral diverticulum formation and persistent chordee. A detailed description of the surgical techniques involved is beyond the scope of this publication and I would refer the reader to the standard operative texts.

Further reading

Bover JG. Current trends in hypospadias repair. *Urology Clinics of North America*, 1999; **26**: 15.
North K, Golding J. A maternal vegetarian diet in pregnancy is associated with hypospadias. The ALSPAC Study Team. Avon Longitudinal Study of Pregnancy and Childhood. *BJU Int*, 2000; **85**: 107–113.
www.pediatrics.org

INTERSEX

Introduction

Disorders of sexual differentiation are the result of abnormalities in the complex process of sexual differentiation which originate on the X and Y chromosomes as well as the autosomes. Sexual determination is dependent on the gonadal type.

Differentiation of the indifferent gonad begins at 6 weeks. The presence of genetic material on the Y chromosome directs the gonad to develop into a testis. The absence of a Y chromosome directs the gonad into the development of an ovary. The testes produce testosterone and Mullerian-inhibiting substance which are important for sexual development and differentiation. Testosterone is converted to its active metabolite dihydrotestosterone (DHT) by 5α reductase.

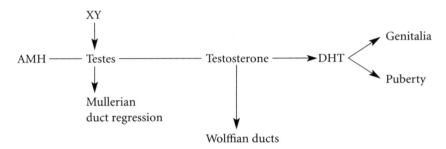

Testosterone stimulates the internal genitalia and Wolffian duct development. The Wolffian ducts in the male form the epididymus, the vas and the seminal vesicles. In the female these structures become Gartners duct at one end and the epoophoron at the other end near the ovary. Mullerian-inhibiting substance also produced by the testes suppresses the Mullerian structures which in the female develop into the fallopian tubes, the uterus and upper third of the vagina. In the male these structures regress to become the appendix testes at one end and the prostatic utricle at the other.

Terminology

Children with ambiguous genitalia are classified as follows:

Virilized Female ——— Hermaphrodite ——— Under-virilized Male

The virilized female is 46XX with ovaries, a female genital tract but virilized external genitalia (e.g. congenital adrenal hyperplasia [CAH]).

The under-virilized male is 46XY with testes and male genital ducts but there is under-virilization of the external genitalia. (e.g. 5α reductase deficiency).

A true hermaphrodite has the presence of both testicular and ovarian tissue. The chromosomal pattern can be 46XX; 46XY or 46XX/XY. There tends to be variable genetic ducts and variable external genitalia.

Aetiology

Congenital adrenal hyperplasia accounts for three-quarters of the virilized 46XX females. This is an autosomal recessive disorder due to a defect in the production of cortisol because of a lack of the enzyme 21-hydroxylase which results in an increase in adrenocorticotrophic hormone ACTH. Males can also be affected.

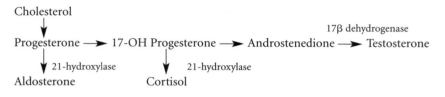

With the severe form of 21-hydroxylase deficiency there is impairment of secretion of both cortisol and aldosterone. This results in electrolyte and fluid losses after the fifth day of life, which are manifested as hyponatraemia, hyperkalaemia, acidosis, dehydration and vascular collapse. Thus, prompt identification of this defect is essential.

Defects in testosterone production (i.e. 17β dehydrogenase) or androgen-dependent target tissues may lead to under-virilization of the male. This is also true for the defects in testosterone metabolism to dihydrotestosterone (DHT) in the peripheral tissues by 5α reductase.

Investigations and management

The inability to confer a sexual gender on a newborn baby can be stressful not only for the parents but also the hospital staff. Prompt recognition and involvement of a specialist at an early stage is essential.

After an examination an initial screen will consist of:

- Karyotype.
- Pelvic ultrasound.
- Renal function and electrolytes.
- 17-OH progesterone.
- Testosterone.
- Gonadotrophins.

This screen will assign the importance of determining the genetic sex and excluding the fatal condition of a salt-losing crisis.

Surgical treatment

In most cases for surgery children are assigned female and any Mullerian remnants excised.

Further reading

Dreger AD. Ambiguous sex or ambivalent medicine – ethical issues in the treatment of intersexuality. *Hastings Cent Rep*, 1988; **28**: 24–35.
Glassberg KI. Gender assignment and the paediatric urologist. *Journal of Urology*, 1999; **161**: 1308–1310.

INTERSTITIAL CYSTITIS

Presentation

Patients present with chronic voiding frequency and bladder pain. They can occasionally pinpoint the day their symptoms started. There may be periods when their symptoms are quiescent.

Demography

The classical patient with interstitial cystitis is a Caucasian female over 40 presenting with a long history of symptoms. Only 10% of cases occur in men. Overall about 10% are classified as severe. A Finnish study estimated the prevalence as 10/100 000 with twice this prevalence in females. A recent study by the NIADDK revealed that women of higher socio-economic status had a higher presentation rate.

Clinical features and diagnosis

As previously mentioned the patients present with irritating lower tract symptoms and bladder pain. They may well have been treated for urinary tract infection intermittently in the community. Upper tract imaging should be normal and the urine sterile and cytology normal. Skene, in 1887, first described the appearance of the bladder in this condition but Hunner has been credited with the description of the classical cystoscopic appearance of severe disease, which is rare (<10%), with large bleeding mucosal ulcers towards the dome of the bladder. In the late 1970s publications by Walsh and Stamey turned the urologist's attention from the hunt for Hunner's ulcer to more subtle changes of mucosal petechial haemorrhage (glomerulation) on decompression and refilling of the bladder at cystoscopy along with the patient's symptom complex. In the late 1980s the NIADDK agreed a research definition of interstitial cystitis along with 18 exclusion criteria. At cystoscopy the bladder should be distended at a pressure of 80 cm (i.e. the irrigation bag 80 cm above bladder level) for 2–3 min and then observed as it empties, haematuria (decompression bleeding) is common and on refilling the classical glomerulations should be present in at least three quadrants of the bladder. It is wise to biopsy the bladder to exclude carcinoma in situ (the microscopic features of IC are not agreed although an undue infiltrate of mast cells is suggestive). In many areas urodynamic evaluation is performed and should show an early first desire to void (hypersensitive) and a relatively low capacity (<350 ml). Recently the instillation of potassium-rich solutions (with subsequent mimicking of symptoms) has been postulated as a diagnostic test.

Aetiology

This is unknown. Theories include an abnormal response to infection, abnormalities of the glycosaminoglycan mucosal barrier, abnormal inflammatory responses (either to stimulus or as an autoimmune disease), neurological abnormalities (sensory and motor) and abnormal urinary constituents. A full discussion of these factors is beyond the scope of this book.

Treatment

As the aetiology is unknown treatment is directed at symptoms. In most centres regular bladder distension under anaesthesia (hydrodistension) is the initial option.

In the UK oral treatment is limited to antihistamines (H1 and H2 receptor antagonists) and analgesics (not non-steroidal anti-inflammatory agents). In the United States Elmiron (sodium pentosan polysulphate) is available; it is said to be excreted in urine and to bolster a deficient mucosal barrier. Intra-vesical treatment with heparin and dimethylsulphoxide (DMSO aka RIMSO) are frequently used with varying response rates and generally require long-term therapy. DMSO has a very offensive smell (personal opinion) and can cause severe halitosis even after one instillation. Numerous other intra-vesical agents have been tried including capsaicin, lignocaine and doxyrubicin with limited efficacy. Referral to pain specialists for TENS machines or acupuncture have also shown limited efficacy. In severe disease which is resistant to all other therapy, surgery in the form of subtotal cystectomy and augmentation cystoplasty or simple ileal loop with or without cystectomy have been reported – it is important to ensure the trigone and urethra are free of IC if augmentation is planned. Pelvic pain has been reported in up to half of patients after these procedures and they can only really be offered as a last resort.

Further reading

Summary of the National Institute of Arthritis. Diabetic, digestive and kidney disease workshop on Interstitial Cystitis. *Journal of Urology*, 1987: **140**: 203–206.

LASERS IN UROLOGY

Advances in lasers and fibreoptics in recent years make them ideally suited to travel through routes in the human body where no hand or scalpel has gone before. With its widespread use of small-diameter endoscopic instruments, urology has been drastically and positively influenced by this technology, perhaps more than any other medical subspecialty.

Laser is an acronym for light amplification by the stimulated emission of radiation. Albert Einstein proposed the concept of stimulated emission of radiation in 1917. It was not until 1960, however, that this theory was put to use by T.H. Maimen to produce the first visible light laser. He used a synthetic ruby crystal with silver-coated ends surrounded by a flash tube to produce light energy. In 1966, Parsons, using a similar ruby laser in a pulsed mode, was the first urologist to experiment with laser light in canine bladders. Mulvany attempted to fragment urinary calculi 2 years later, again using the ruby laser.

By adding electricity, heat or light energy to atoms in their ground state, their energy level can be raised. The energy is then released spontaneously in the form of photons or electromagnetic (EM) waves to return to the ground state. When a photon of light energy of the same wavelength strikes an excited atom, that photon and the photon of light that is released are discharged simultaneously and therefore will be identical in frequency and phase. This is the concept of stimulated emission used in the creation of a laser. Atoms in their ground state undergo absorption of photons of light energy. For stimulated emission to occur, more atoms must exist in the excited state than in the ground state, a situation known as a population inversion. Energy must be supplied to this population. In a laser, the energy source is usually electric or flashlamp driven. The populations of atoms or molecules that become excited are the lasing medium.

The three characteristics mentioned above differentiate laser light from natural light. These are coherence (the photons are all in phase), collimation (they travel parallel with no divergence), and monochromaticity (they all have the same wavelength and, therefore, the same colour if within the visible light spectrum).

Different lasing mediums (which can be either solid, liquid or gas) emit photons in different wavelengths of the EM spectrum. This is at least partly responsible for the unique characteristics of a particular laser.

The biophysics of laser–tissue interactions

Local tissue properties, combined with the wavelength of laser light used, further affect the quality of the laser–tissue interaction. Examples of tissue properties include the density, degree of opacity (e.g. quantity of pigments), water content and blood supply of the tissue. The more dense or opaque a tissue is, the greater the degree of absorption of light energy and the greater the degree of transformation to heat.

Molecules, proteins and pigments may absorb light only in a specific range of wavelengths. Haemoglobin, for example, absorbs light energy that has a wavelength as high as 600 nm and is translucent to light beyond this range. (The argon laser produces light of 458–515 nm and, therefore, is heavily absorbed by haemoglobin.) Water also absorbs in a specific wavelength range, beginning with a small amount of absorption from 300–2000 nm, at which point the degree of absorption increases rapidly and continues for several thousand nanometers. The CO_2 laser produces light in the far infrared spectrum, at 10600 nm. This is heavily absorbed by water contained in tissue and, therefore, does not penetrate deeply.

Local blood circulation affects the degree of laser energy absorption via two mechanisms. First, as mentioned above, the absorptive properties of individual blood components (e.g. haemoglobin, water) differ and interact with light in specific wavelength ranges. Secondly, the circulating blood acts as a heat sink or radiator by transporting absorbed thermal energy away from the site of delivery. This effectively blunts laser power by opposing its local thermal effects.

The wavelength of laser light can be proportional to the depth of penetration into specific tissues. The longer the wavelength, the deeper the expected penetration. Tissue composition and molecular absorption is among several other factors that play into the laser end effect. The neodymium:yttrium-aluminium-garnet (Nd:YAG) laser, for example, produces light in the near infrared region (1060 nm) and penetrates to a depth of approximately 5–10 mm in most tissues (at its wavelength, Nd:YAG is not absorbed by haemoglobin or water in any significant quantity). The CO_2 laser with a wavelength of 10600 nm (a longer wavelength, thus should penetrate more deeply) only penetrates to a depth of less than 0.1 mm because its wavelength is very highly absorbed by tissue water. Ultimately, laser energy and tissue characteristics interact in a complex manner that determines the degree of absorption, penetration, reflection and scattering of laser energy.

Surgeons currently using lasers seek four different effects – thermal, mechanical, photochemical and tissue welding effects (which is actually mediated through thermal energy). The most common utilization is the thermal effect, whereby light energy is absorbed and transformed into heat. This results in the denaturation of proteins at 42–65°C, the shrinkage of arteries and veins at 70°C and cellular dehydration at 100°C. Once water has completely evaporated from tissue, a rapid rise in temperature ensues, carbonization then occurs at 250°C, and, finally, vaporization occurs at 300°C.

The mechanical effect results, for example, when a very high power density is directed at a urinary calculus and a column of electrons is freed rapidly at the stone surface. This creates a plasma bubble that swiftly expands and acts like a sonic boom to disrupt the stone along stress lines.

The photochemical effect refers to the selective activation of a specific drug or molecule, which may be administered systemically but is taken up in selected tissues. By activation of the molecule or drug by a specific wavelength of light, the molecule is transformed into a toxic compound(s), often involving oxygen-free radicals that can cause cellular death through destruction of DNA cross-links. This is a novel approach to destroying superficial skin or mucosal malignant and pre-malignant lesions. Lasers are ideally suited because of their power and specific wavelength. Finally, the tissue-welding effect is derived by focusing light of a particular wavelength to induce collagen cross-linking. By adding proteinaceous materials (e.g. 50% human albumin, also known as tissue solder) directly to the tissue edges to be welded or a chromophore that absorbs at the laser's wavelength, one can achieve an increased tensile strength.

Laser types and clinical applications

1. CO_2 laser. The CO_2 laser emits in the invisible far infrared portion of the EM spectrum, at 10600 nm. It usually is coupled with a visible helium-neon beam for guidance. Its beam is highly absorbed by water; therefore, it vaporizes water-dense tissues to a superficial depth of less than 1 mm. Heat conduction results in thermal coagulation down to a depth of about 0.5 mm, with only small vessels less than 0.5 mm coagulated effectively.

2. Neodymium:yttrium-aluminium-garnet laser. The ND:YAG laser emits a beam at 1064 nm (near infrared) and can be delivered in a continuous, pulsed or Q-switched mode. The 1064 nm wavelength allows for a relatively deep penetration of as much as 10 mm because this frequency is outside the absorption peaks of both haemoglobin and water. It has good haemostatic (coagulates blood vessels as much as 5 mm in diameter) and cutting properties and also is suitable for lithotripsy when Q-switched.

An optical fibre is employed for delivery, which may be passed through all types of endoscopes. A sapphire or crystal tip may also be used at the end of an optical fibre, which decreases backscatter and allows for precise cutting using a direct touch technique.

3. Potassium-titanyl phosphate crystal laser. This laser, also known as a KTP laser, yields a green visible light beam of 532 nm by passing an Nd:YAG-produced beam (1064 nm) through a KTP crystal that doubles its frequency (thus, halves its wavelength). This light penetrates less than Nd:YAG because of its shorter wavelength and its absorption by haemoglobin. It is used for incisions, resection and ablation and can be passed through an optical fibre and thus through endoscopic instruments. One disadvantage of KTP laser energy is that tissue carbonization can be observed, rather than a true ablative effect.

4. Dye lasers. The lasing medium is an organic liquid dye that must be excited optically by another laser or flash lamp. The wavelength emitted depends on the type of dye used, which can be changed or adjusted. The emitted light, therefore, can be tuned to cover a wide spectrum of visible light. In the pulsed mode, this laser is used for lithotripsy and ablation of vascular lesions. The most common dye employed is coumarin, which produces a wavelength of 504 nm when excited by a flashlamp. As opposed to a solid-state laser, the dye in the lasing chamber requires replacement, which may be inconvenient and expensive compared with the maintenance of newer laser systems.

5. Holmium:YAG laser. Holmium:YAG (Ho:YAG) is a more recent addition. It consists of the rare earth element holmium, doped in a YAG crystal that emits a beam of 2150 nm. This laser energy is delivered most commonly in a pulsatile manner, using a thermo-mechanical mechanism of action. It superheats water, which heavily absorbs light energy at this wavelength. This creates a vaporization bubble at the tip of a low-water density quartz or silica fibre used for delivery. This vapour bubble expands rapidly and destabilizes the molecules it contacts. This is ideal for lithotripsy of all stone types. The absorption depth in tissue is 1–2 mm, as long as it is employed in a water-based medium. This specific light energy provides good haemostasis when used in a pulsed mode of 250 ms duration and at low pulse repetition rate. It also may be used for incisions at higher repetition rates.

6. Summary of laser types and current clinical applications

- For soft tissue incisions (e.g. urethral strictures, posterior urethral valves, endopyelotomy, bladder neck contractures), use Ho:YAG, Nd:YAG, or KTP.
- For resection and ablation (e.g. benign prostatic hyperplasia [BPH], TCC, condylomata, penile carcinoma, bladder and skin haemangiomata), use Nd:YAG, Ho:YAG, KTP:YAG, or CO_2.
- For lithotripsy (renal pelvis, ureter and bladder stones), use Ho:YAG, or pulsed dye.
- For tissue welding (e.g. vasovasotomy; urethral reconstruction for hypospadias, strictures, diverticula, or fistulas; pyeloplasty, bladder augmentation, and continent urinary diversion), use KTP, Nd:YAG, or CO_2.

MALE INFERTILITY

Introduction

Infertility is defined as the inability of a couple to conceive after one year of unprotected intercourse. Fifteen percent of couples experience reproductive difficulty. It appears that 50% is due to a male factor problem and 50% to female issues.

The testicles have the dual function of spermatogenesis, which occurs in the seminiferous tubules, and secretion of the male steroid hormones from the Leydig cells. These mechanisms are under the control of the hypothalamic–pituitary–gonadal axis and are required for the development of normal secondary sexual characteristics and reproduction.

Hormonal control and spermatogenesis

The seminiferous tubules contain germ cells at various stages of maturation and Sertoli cells; these account for 85–90% of testicular volume. The Sertoli cells are a fixed population of support cells and appear to be involved in the nourishment of developing germ cells and phagocytosis of damaged cells. The spermatogenic (germinal cells) are arranged in an orderly manner from the basement membrane to the lumen. Spermatogonia lie directly on the basement membrane and, next in order, progressing centrally, are found primary spermatocytes, secondary spermatocytes and spermatids. These are the precursor developmental stages for spermatozoa.

The hypothalamic–pituitary–gonadal axis is a closed loop feedback control mechanism. Luteinizing hormone (LH) and follicular stimulating hormone (FSH) are synthesized in the anterior pituitary gland and secreted in response to the episodic release of gonadotrophin-releasing hormone (GnRH) from the hypothalamus. LH has a direct effect on the Leydig cells to produce testosterone. Sertoli cells and the seminiferous tubules are the target for FSH, and thus required for the initiation of spermatogenesis.

Assessment

The most effective and efficient way to investigate and manage couples with infertility is to see them jointly with a gynaecologist. This enables a coordinated assessment of investigations and prevents unnecessary tests.

A careful medical/sexual history and examination of the male partner provides part of the initial consultation. Two semen analyses and blood for haematology, routine biochemistry and a hormonal profile (FSH, LH, prolactin, testosterone) are taken.

History

A good understanding of the causes of male infertility is important when documenting the history and clinical examination. Developmental abnormalities are important. Delayed puberty may indicate the presence of Klinefelter's syndrome. Previous bladder neck or pelvic surgical procedures may cause retrograde ejaculation. Infections involving the urogenital tract may cause testicular damage or obstruction to the reproductive ducts. Even a severe febrile illness can cause impairment to spermatogenesis. Testicular failure may also result from previous trauma, following hernia repair and torsion. The semen parameters can be affected by toxins such as tobacco, recreational drugs, alcohol and pharmaceutical agents, that is, cimetidine, anabolic steroids, sulfasalazine, spironolactone or previous treatment with chemotherapy.

Physical examination

The examination should pay particular attention to body development and secondary sexual characteristics which may indicate a hormonal or chromosomal cause for infertility.

Testicular examination is extremely important as approximately 95% of testicular volume is made up of seminiferous tubules. A Prader orchidometer may be used to assess testicular size. A volume generally greater than 15 ml indicates normal spermatogenesis. Penile abnormalities such as hypospadias and phimosis may cause problems of deposition of semen within the female genital tract. Congenital bilateral absence of the vas deferens (CBAVD) and thus obstructive azoospermia is associated with cystic fibrosis. The female partners of CBAVD patients should be routinely assessed for mutations in the cystic fibrosis gene and councilled appropriately.

The presence of a varicocele can affect the semen parameters and in uncontrolled studies varicocele repair resulted in pregnancy rates of 30–40%.

Interpretation of results and investigations

Standardization of the guidelines for collection and assessment of semen analysis has been provided by the World Health Organization (WHO).

Semen analysis

Samples should be collected by masturbation into a sterile container after at least 3 days of abstinence. More than one sample should be obtained over a 3-month or greater time span as counts can be variable and be affected by a number of factors as outlined in the history. The presence of inflammatory cells may indicate an underlying urinary infection or prostatitis. Anti-sperm antibodies (IgA, IgG) are present in approximately 10% of infertile men. These antibodies may occur secondary to a testicular insult. Treatment of this condition with steroids remains controversial, but some studies have suggested improved pregnancy rates.

1. **Volume.** >2 ml.

2. **Density.** 20 million per ml. A sample of <10 million per ml indicates subfertility.

3. **Motility.** >50% motile.

4. **Morphology.** At least 50% need to be intact mature sperm. This is the best overall predictor of fertility.

Hormonal analysis

When the semen analysis indicates azoospermia, FSH and LH results allow the discrimination between primary testicular failure and obstructive azoospermia.

An FSH and LH >10 units indicates primary testicular failure. A result of >30 would suggest a less than 10% chance of ongoing spermatogenesis.

If the FSH and LH are normal then azoospermia is likely to be due to obstruction. Treatment may therefore be instigated depending on clinical and radiological findings. The use of transrectal ultrasound (TRUS) may indicate the site of obstruction, that is, ejaculatory duct cyst which may be amenable to endoscopic surgery.

Hyperprolactinaemia is associated with oligospermia.

Chromosomal/genetic abnormalities

There are well-recognized genetic causes for male infertility such as Klinefelter's syndrome (sex chromosome aneuploidy). Approximately 10% of patients with an unknown cause of infertility have an abnormal karyotype. This has implications for genetic counselling prior to assisted conception.

It is also now known that men with azoospermia have deletions of the long arm of the Y chromosome (azoospermia factor AZF). Gene mapping has identified the 'Deleted in azoospermia gene' (DAZ). The importance of this finding is such that, in obstructive azoospermia, the clinician may be able to identify patients with focal spermatogenesis which can be harvested for an ICSI (intra-cytoplasmic sperm injection) programme.

Assisted conception

The advent of techniques such as ICSI have completely revolutionized the treatment of male factor infertility. This involves the direct injection of a spermatozoa into an ovum to achieve fertilization. The success of this technique is approximately 20–25% per cycle of treatment.

Sperm aspiration

For patients with obstructed azoospermia, sperm retrieval and freezing is available. Sperm may be aspirated percutaneously directly from the epididymus under local or general anaesthetic (PESA – percutaneous sperm aspiration). If this is unsuccessful then through a scrotal incision the testes can be delivered and epididymal tubules identified with the aid of an operating microscope and seminal fluid then aspirated. An embryologist needs to be present in theatre to confirm the presence of motile spermatozoa and store samples (MESA – microscopic sperm aspiration).

There is now no place for isolated testicular biopsy, but samples of testicular tissue can be snap frozen and motile sperm teased out (TESE – testicular sperm aspiration). In the presence of focal testicular spermatogenesis, multiple testicular biopsies may be required.

Conclusions

Our understanding of the causes for male factor infertility and techniques such as ICSI has completely changed our understanding and approach to this condition. In the future we may well be able to identify specific genetic defects and treat with targeted genetic therapies.

Further reading

Jequier A. *Male Infertility: A Guide for the Clinician*. Oxford: Blackwell Publishers, 2000.

METABOLIC STONE DISEASE

Stone composition

The majority of urinary stones in the western world are composed of calcium in combination with oxalate (70–80%), phosphate (5–10%), uric acid and struvite (magnesium ammonium phosphate) accounting for 5–10% each and rare amino acid (cysteine, xantheine) or drug therapy (indinavir, triamterine) stones the remainder.

Stone formation

Normal urine is supersaturated with solute. Several factors prevent solute precipitation leading to stone formation.

The principal factor is probably the continuous flow of urine with inhibitory ions (citrate, magnesium) and urinary proteins (e.g. Tamm–Horsfall protein, prothrombin fragment 1) having additional inhibitory effects. Stones usually form on a surface, for example, epithelial cell, red blood cell (nucleation), and then further aggregation occurs. Stasis allows prolonged exposure of the nascent calculus to supersaturated urine and predisposes to infection.

Predisposing factors to stone formation are:

- Low fluid intake
- Urinary tract abnormality (e.g. PUJ obstruction)
- Urinary tract infection
- Foreign bodies
- Hypercalcaemia (hyperparathyroidism, etc.)
- Hyperuricaemia (gout, myeloproliferative disorders)
- Defects in renal tubular function (renal tubular acidosis)
- Defects of amino acid transport (cysteinuria)
- Dietary factors
  (i)   High sodium/sugar intake
  (ii) High animal protein intake
  (iii) High oxalate intake.

Metabolic assessment

1. Why? With no attempt at prevention all stone formers will make another stone, 40% will have re-formed stone within 3 years and virtually all patients after 25 years. This has financial implications – from the direct cost of investigation/intervention and also the indirect cost to society of the patient's absence from work.

2. Who?

Low recurrence risk patients (limited screen)	High recurrence risk patients (complete screen)
Single stone No anatomical defects Sterile urine	Children and young adults Strong family history Gout Inflammatory bowel disease Nephrocalcinosis Abnormal limited screen

3. When? The optimum time to investigate this group of patients is after an acute attack of pain. They are far more likely to comply with the investigations at this point and, if therapy is indicated, comply with the regimen.

4. How?

- Limited screen

Stone analysis	Stone composition will target any further investigations
Serum analysis	Urea and electrolytes, creatinine, calcium, magnesium, phosphate, urate
Urinanalysis	Dipstick, culture and first void pH (cysteine spot test)
Dietary assessment	Fluid intake Salt/sugar Animal/dairy protein Oxalate rich food (nuts, spinach, tea, broccoli) Fibre
Clinical history	Occupation, medication, past history

- Complete screen

All aspects of the limited screen plus:

Serum analysis	Parathyroid hormone, Vitamin D
Urine (2 24-h collections)	1. Volume, calcium, phosphate, magnesium, oxalate, sodium, citrate, creatinine (acid container) 2. Volume, pH, urate and cysteine (if spot test positive) plain container
Further urinary tests as dictated by above	1. 24-h calcium with dietary restriction 2. Calcium load testing 3. Acid load test

Intervention

The primary intervention in all stone formers is to encourage an adequate fluid intake – at least 4 pints of water in addition to their current intake. A useful method is to recommend drinking a 500-ml size bottle of water with every meal and one over the course of the morning and afternoon.

Specific investigations

- Blood abnormality

Hypercalcaemia	Serum PTH (hyperparathyroidism, hypothyroid) Thyroid function (hyper- or hypothyroid); Chest X-ray (primary or metastatic cancer, sarcoid, TB); Further investigation/intervention dependent on the above
Renal failure	Estimation of GFR (creatinine clearance or isotope methods) Referral to nephrologist if no surgically correctable cause (i.e. renal obstruction or persistent calculi)
Hyperuricaemia	Consider therapy with allopurinol

- Urinary abnormality

Low volume	Encourage oral intake
Infection	Clear stone burden, antibiotic prophylaxis until sterile mid-stream specimen of urine on at least two occasions (3 months minimum)
Hypercalciuria	If due to hypercalcaemia as above check fasting/loading urinary calcium Initial fluid advice, dependent on classification Therapy with thiazides, potassium citrate or phosphate supplements
Hyperuricosuria	Consider therapy with allopurinol (if patient has gout) Fluid advice Potassium citrate supplements (may dissolve stone)
Hypocitraturia	Potassium citrate supplements Fresh lemonade
Cysteinuria	Fluid advice (3000 ml/day) Alkalinize urine (potassium citrate) Binding agents (penicillamine, captopril)

Further reading

Campbell MF, Retik AB, Darracott Vaughan E, Walsh PC. *Campbell's Urology*. 7th edn. WB Saunders Co, 1997.

Robertson WG. Medical management of urinary stone disease. *European Urology Update Series*. 1998; **7**: 139–144.

Ryall RL. The scientific basis of calcium oxalate stone formation. In: Mundy AR, Fitzpatrick J, Neal D, eds. *The Scientific Basis of Urology*. Oxford: Isis Medical Media, 1999.

PELVIURETERIC JUNCTION OBSTRUCTION

Presentation

1. Prenatal

- Routine use of ultrasonography in pregnancy and particularly second trimester scans can identify hydronephrosis.
- An a–p diameter of the foetal renal pelvis greater than 1 cm suggests obstruction.
- Management is expectant and investigation is initiated postpartum.
- PUJ obstruction accounts for 80% of prenatally diagnosed hydronephrosis.

2. Incidental

- Child or adult during investigation of non-urological symptoms.

3. Symptomatic

- Episodic loin pain.
- Haematuria (both micro and macroscopic).
- Pyuria or infection (possibly pyonephrosis).
- Occasionally the patient may present in renal failure if the disease is bilateral or present in a solitary kidney.
- The dilated pelvis is more vulnerable to traumatic rupture.

Demography

- Bilateral obstruction occurs in approximately 15% of cases.
- Hydronephrosis is present in <1% of live births.
- 2.5 times more common in males.
- 2.5 times more common on the left side.

Aetiology

1. Primary. The aetiology of PUJ obstruction is still controversial. Incomplete canalization during ureterogenesis along with abnormal development or orientation of the smooth muscle layers of the ureteral wall have been advanced as theories of obstruction intrinsic to the ureteric wall. Extrinsic obstruction is frequently attributed to a lower pole vessel passing anterior to the ureter of pelviureteric junction. This vessel is often described as aberrant, but is a variation of normal present in a minority of the population but present in around one-third of patients with PUJ obstruction.

2. Secondary

- After stone passage.
- Trauma (iatrogenic).
- Ureteric tumour.
- High-grade vesicoureteric obstruction.
- After previous pyeloplasty.

Differential diagnosis

1. Prenatal

- Megaureter.
- Vesicoureteric reflux (primary or secondary to posterior urethral valves).

2. Childhood

- Wilms tumour.
- Neuroblastoma.
- Polycystic or multicystic kidney.

3. Adult

- Renal cell cancer.
- Other retroperitoneal tumour or nodal disease.
- Ureteric tumour.
- Stones.
- Ureteric stricture (benign, malignant, TB).

Diagnosis and management

- Ultrasound.
- Intravenous urogram
    (i)   To delineate anatomy (large renal pelvis/caliectasis with no ureteric filling or normal calibre ureter).
- Diuretic renography.
    (i)   Technetium 99 DTPA or Tc MAG 3.
    (ii) Frusemide is given either 20 min after isotope injection (F+20) or 15 min (F−15) before will give a definitive diagnosis of obstruction and also provide information on divided renal function.
    (iii) Frusemide provides its maximal effect around 18 min after injection as such an F+20 renogram will demonstrate obstruction late on in the investigation and may give equivocal results.
    (iv) The F−15 renogram provides maximal stress (in terms of flow) on the PUJ early in the investigation and if economic or logistic problems may prevent multiple investigations is the renogram of choice.
- Retrograde ureterography.
    (i)   If the ureter has never been demonstrated, to show normal calibre.
    (ii) Optimal timing controversial.
- Early risk of infection in closed system/chemical pyelitis.
- Late risk of missing ureteric pathology.
- Diagnostic ureteroscopy.
    (i)   Endoluminal ultrasound scan to assess for crossing vessels.
    (ii) Ureteric stenting to facilitate later ureteroscopy.
- Contrast CT angiography.
    (i)   To assess the presence and site of any crossing vessels.

Management

1. ### *Minimally invasive*

- Contraindications.
  - (i) Significant dilatation of the pelvis (>30 cc).
  - (ii) Poor renal function.
  - (iii) Crossing vessels.
- Balloon dilatation (endoburst).
  - (i) Cystoscopy and retrograde pyelography to delineate the PUJ.
  - (ii) Balloon dilatation catheter is passed through the stenosis.
  - (iii) Dilatation to 16 Fr waisting of the balloon is usually noted.
  - (iv) Extravasation after loss of waist is a good sign.
  - (v) Ureteric stent for 6 weeks.
  - (vi) Success in 67% with long-term follow-up.
- Endopyelotomy.
- Retrograde.
  - (i) Cystoscopy and retrograde pyelography to delineate the PUJ.
  - (ii) Flexible or rigid ureteroscopy (with safety guidewire).
  - (iii) Incision with electrocautery or holmium laser.
  - (iv) Incision classically posterolaterally to avoid crossing vessels (or if endo-luminal ultrasound available away from vessels).
  - (v) Balloon dilatation to confirm disruption and extravasation.
  - (vi) Ureteric stent post-operatively (6–8 weeks).
  - (vii) Best series 87.5% pain free and unobstructed (mean follow-up 10 months).
- Antegrade.
  - (i) Percutaneous puncture after retrograde pyelography.
  - (ii) Preferably through upper or middle calyx.
  - (iii) PUJ incised with electrocautery, laser or cold knife.
  - (iv) Posterolateral incision (dependent on CT angiogram).
  - (v) Specific endopyelotomy stent (14 Fr tapering to 8.2 or 7 Fr).
  - (vi) Best series 85% pain free and unobstructed.
- Laparoscopic.
  - (i) Transperitoneal or retroperitoneal route.
  - (ii) Requires advanced laparoscopic skills.
  - (iii) Intracorporeal suturing of anastamosis.
  - (iv) Appears equivalent to open surgery in the short term.
  - (v) Shorter hospital stay and convalescence.

2. ### *Maximally invasive*

- Open pyeloplasty.
  - (i) The current gold standard.
  - (ii) Long-term follow-up available (first described in 1911).
  - (iii) Many techniques described.
  - (iv) The aim is to remodel the PUJ into a wide funnel shape.
  - (v) Dismembered pyeloplasty (Hynes–Anderson).
    - PUJ excised.
    - Ureter spatulated.

- Reduction of renal pelvis volume.
- Anastomosis with absorbable stitch.
- Stent or nephrostomy drainage.
  (vi) 96% success rates at 10 years.
- Nephrectomy.
  (i) Laparoscopic or open procedure.
  (ii) Treatment of choice in the poorly functioning (<10%) renal unit.
  (iii) Decompression and repeat renogram in 3 months indicated if global loss of renal function.

Further reading

Bagley D *et al.* Ureteroscopic treatment of ureteropelvic junction obstruction. *Journal of Urology*, 1998; **160**: 1643–1647.

Djurhuus *et al.* Pelviureteric dynamics. *European Urology Update Series*, 1997; **6**: 21–26.

Eden CG *et al.* Laparoscopic dismembered pyeloplasty: 50 consecutive cases. *BJU Int*, 2001; **88**: 526–531.

Jabbour ME, Goldfischer ER, Klima WJ, Stravodimos KG, Smith AD. Endopyelotomy after failed pyeloplasty: the long-term results. *Journal of Urology*, 1998; **160**: 690–692.

O'Reilly PH *et al.* The long-term results of Anderson-Hynes pyeloplasty. *BJU Int*, 2001; **87**: 287–289.

Van Cangh *et al.* Endourological management of pelviureteric junction obstruction: Endoureteropyelotomy. *European Urology Update Series*, 1997; **6**: 1–7.

Webber RJ, Pardian SS, McClinton S, Hussey J. Retrograde balloon dilatation for pelviureteric junction obstruction: long-term follow-up. *Journal of Endourology*, 1997; **11**: 239–242.

PENILE AND GENITAL TRAUMA

Major penile trauma is relatively rare. The commonest injury is undoubtedly superficial skin trauma from zippers or frenular lacerations during intercourse. Occasionally these may require exploration and suture under anaesthesia. Repair should be performed with absorbable sutures such as vicryl. Penile amputation is rare and may be the result of assault, self-harm or trauma. Repair is best performed by surgeons experienced in microvascular anastomotic techniques and nerve repair and in most UK centres referral to a plastic surgeon is the most appropriate course of action.

Penile fracture

Aetiology

Penile trauma occurs most commonly during sexual activity, be this masturbation or vigorous intercourse, with only about 30% of injuries occurring in other situations (e.g. direct trauma or during sleep). Ninety-eight percent of fractures occur with an erect penis. Approximately 10% of fractures are associated with a urethral injury – in this event haematuria or blood at the meatus will be noted.

Symptoms and signs

The classical scenario is of an audible crack followed by immediate detumescence and a rapid onset of penile bruising. Occasionally the patient may present at a later stage having noticed pain during intercourse and later developing penile angulation.

Differential diagnosis

1. Rupture of dorsal vein of penis.
2. Rupture of dorsal artery.
3. Rupture of suspensory ligament.

Investigation

Clinical examination is usually hampered by pain. Cavernosography will reveal extravasation of contrast. Some authors have suggested ultrasound to visualize the tear.

Management

Immediate surgical exploration is the treatment of choice and is associated with potency rates of 97%. A coronal type incision +/− circumcision and degloving of the penis usually allows adequate exposure to evacuate haematoma and then repair the corpora with an absorbable suture such as vicryl. If there is associated urethral injury the edges should be freshened and closed with an absorbable suture. It is best to insert either a urethral or suprapubic catheter and cover the procedure with a broad-spectrum antibiotic.

Ruptured suspensory ligament

Symptoms

- Pain/bruising.
- Floating penis (i.e. abnormal position during erection).

Management

This is by exploration and repair via an infrapubic incision.

Scrotal and testicular trauma

Injury can be either blunt or penetrating.

Symptoms and signs

Pain is likely, but thorough clinical examination will demonstrate the presence (or absence) of a scrotal haematoma and a palpable testis.

Investigation

If the testicle is impalpable (or pain too severe) ultrasonography may help delineate the testis.

Management

Lacerations and penetrating trauma require exploration and wound toilet. If the testis is intact but contused scrotal support and analgesia along with bed rest is usually all that is needed. If there is a large haematocele or the testis is disrupted again exploration is required. A mid-line raphe incision is utilized and any haematocele evacuated. Necrotic seminiferous tubules are excised and the tunica albergina repaired with a running non-absorbable suture. Dartos and skin are closed with absorbable suture material. It is always wise to obtain consent for orchidectomy and advise the patient that the testicle may become atrophic. If the testicle is beyond repair orchidectomy should be performed. Drains are best avoided and the procedure should be covered with a broad-spectrum antibiotic.

PRIAPISM

Priapism is a prolonged erection, occurring in the absence of sexual stimulation and is not relieved by orgasm. It is uncommon, but seen more frequently following the introduction of treatment for erectile dysfunction. There is no identifiable cause in 60% of patients while the remaining 40% are associated with a secondary cause. These include leukaemia, pelvic malignancy, pelvic infections, penile trauma, spinal cord injury or the use of medications.

Presentation

The patient usually presents with a history of several hours of a painful erection. Eighty percent occur during sleep or following sexual activity (17%). The erection involves the cavernosal bodies but not the glans penis or the corpus spongiosum. Priapism represents a urological emergency and requires prompt treatment, to avoid impotence resulting from thrombosis damaging the erectile tissue.

Classification

1. High flow (non-ischaemic). This is due to penile or perineal trauma and results when injury creates an arterial–sinusoidal shunt within the corpus cavernosum. It is uncommon.

2. Low flow (ischaemic). Many cases have no known aetiology. This is the most frequent cause and results in persistent cavernosal relaxation. Drugs can cause a low flow priapism by different mechanisms. Psychotropic agents may have peripheral α-blocking activity or central serotonin-like activity. Intra-cavernous pharmacotherapy is a technique used to treat erectile dysfunction. Drugs are commonly injected into the corporal bodies to produce an erection. These include prostaglandin E1, phentolamine (α-blocker) or papaverine (phosphodiesterase inhibitor).

Investigations

A full history and haematological analysis is required. If there is doubt as to the classification of the priapism then a blood gas analysis should be performed. If the presence of a high flow priapism is suspected colour duplex ultrasound and arteriography will be necessary for diagnosis and subsequent treatment by means of embolization.

Management

1. High flow. A high flow priapism is treated with pudendal arteriography with embolization. Open ligation of abnormal vessels may sometimes be required. The use of digoxin has also been recommended.

2. Low flow. Non-operative treatment should always be the first line of treatment. A 19-gauge butterfly is inserted into one of the corporal bodies and blood aspirated (this can be sent for blood gas analysis). This process continues until the aspirate is bright red. If unsuccessful the corporal body can be irrigated with an α-agonist (10 mg phenylephrine in 500 ml saline). This can be continued every 10–15 min until the erection subsides.

If these options fail then surgical treatment is required to establish a shunt between the erect corporal body and the glans penis, or corpus spongiosum, or saphenous vein.

Outcome

Priapism will recur in 10–60% especially if the aetiology is idiopathic or due to sickle cell disease. Impotence will occur in about 10–40% but will be increased if a surgical intervention has been performed.

PROSTATIC CARCINOMA (CaP)

Any discussion of prostate cancer needs to begin with the acknowledgement that this is perhaps the area of greatest controversy in urology. These controversies stem from the fact that the incidence of prostate cancer is high in older men. However, some would argue that these men die 'with not of' prostate cancer. There is therefore concern amongst some that early diagnosis and radical treatment of prostate cancer has the potential for marked over-treatment, without significant benefit in survival or quality of life. The opposing argument would maintain that early diagnosis and radical treatment improves survival. It is not the scope of this chapter to deal with this controversy, but it is impossible to deal with CaP without acknowledging it.

Epidemiology

In most Western countries CaP is the commonest male cancer in middle age and beyond. It is now second only to lung cancer as a cause of cancer deaths in men. There has been a significant increase in the incidence of the disease over the past decade. It is estimated that the lifetime risk of a man developing microscopic foci of CaP is 30%, clinically significant CaP 10% and the risk of dying from CaP is 3%.

Risk factors

- Age. Clinical disease is rare in those below 50.
- Race. Incidence is higher in North America and northern Europe. Within the USA the risk is higher within black populations than in white.
- Genetic. There is a two- to threefold increase in men with a first-degree relative who has CaP.
- Diet. There is a correlation between high fat, high protein diets and CaP.

Diagnosis

1. Symptoms. Although most CaPs arise in the periphery of the gland, symptoms of CaP often mimic identically those of benign prostatic hyperplasia, which occurs in the transitional zone.

2. Digital rectal examination (DRE). The diagnosis may be suspected from the hard nodular feel of the prostate. Accuracy of this is 30–50%.

3. PSA testing. Over the last decade the use of Prostate Specific Antigen to test for CaP has become common (normal values 0–4 ng/ml). This protease is secreted almost exclusively by the prostate and, although often thought of as a marker for CaP, can in fact be elevated in a number of conditions such as urinary retention, urinary tract infection, prostatitis, and after instrumentation such as catheterization or cystoscopy. The PSA test unfortunately lacks specificity. As a result, a number of refinements have been introduced to try to improve the specificity of the test:

- Age-related PSA. Differing normal values depending on decade of life.
- PSA density. Relating level to size of prostate.
- PSA velocity. Measuring the rate of rise of PSA rather than a single value.

- Free/total PSA. Relating the bound PSA to the free level in the serum.

Although all these variations offer some advantage, none has solved the problem of the lack of specificity of PSA as a marker.

4. Transrectal ultrasound and biopsy (TRUS). Because of this lack of specificity further tests are needed to try to make the diagnosis of CaP. Ultrasound of the prostate transrectally offers the ability not only to assess the prostatic margins but to guide biopsies to any abnormal areas of the gland. Biopsies are necessary because the ultrasound appearances of CaP are not diagnostic. This test is currently the gold standard for the diagnosis of CaP but even this carries a 25% false-negative rate. In addition, it carries the risk of morbidity from infection and must be covered with antibiotic prophylaxis.

5. Screening. Because of the above problems with diagnosis and the concerns about the necessity/benefit of treatment, the case for screening for prostate cancer using DRE and PSA testing remains unproven. There is an ongoing Europe-wide screening study to try to answer this question.

Stage and grade

1. Stage. CaP is staged using the UICC TNM classification:

- Primary tumour
- T1 Tumour impalpable
  - T1a incidental finding in <5% of all tissue resected at TURP
  - T1b incidental finding in >5% of all tissue resected at TURP
  - T1c tumour identified by needle biopsy because of raised PSA
- T2 Tumour confined within the prostate
  - T2a tumour involves one lobe only
  - T2b tumour involves both lobes
- T3 Tumour extends through the prostatic capsule.
  - T3a tumour extends through capsule unilaterally or bilaterally
  - T3b tumour involves seminal vesicles.
- T4 Tumour is fixed or invades adjacent structures other than seminal vesicles.

- Nodal disease
- Nx regional nodes cannot be assessed
- N0 no regional lymph node metastases
- N1 regional lymph node metastases.

- Metastatic disease
- Mx status not known
- M0 no metastatic disease
- M1 metastatic disease present.
- M1a non regional lymph nodes
- M1b bony metastases
- M1c metastases in other sites.

2. Grade. CaP is graded using a scoring system known as the Gleason Score. This recognizes five grades according to histological pattern.

- Grade 1 small uniform glands with minimal nuclear changes.
- Grade 2 medium sized acini with stromal separation.
- Grade 3 variation in glandular size with infiltration of stroma.
- Grade 4 extensive infiltration and cytological atypia.
- Grade 5 sheets of undifferentiated cancer cells.

The pathologist assesses the two most prominent areas of grades and these numbers are added together to give the Gleason Score (between 2 and 10). This is often broadly grouped together:

- <4 Well differentiated
- 5–7 Moderately differentiated
- >7 Poorly differentiated

Patterns of spread

CaP tends to spread locally and to regional lymph nodes and by blood-borne spread to bone.

- Staging of local disease is done routinely by PSA testing, DRE and TRUS. CT scanning and MRI have been advocated but neither is sufficiently reliable to assure organ confined disease.
- Metastatic disease is staged most usefully by radionucleotide bone scan. This investigation is thought to be unnecessary in those men with a PSA of < 15 ng/ml in the absence of symptoms.

Management

The treatment of CaP is controversial. Obviously the treatment options depend on whether the disease is confined to the prostate.

- Management of localized disease.
- Active monitoring. Regular clinical review and monitoring of PSA. Institution of treatment dependent on symptoms and +/− rising PSA.

1. Radiotherapy. This can be given by external beam or by interstitial seed implantation (brachytherapy).

2. Radical prostatectomy. This involves removal of the entire prostate gland and anastomosis of the bladder neck to the urethra. It can be performed by either the retropubic approach or the perineal approach and has more recently been performed laparoscopically.

This procedure should be restricted to those with disease localized to the prostate, a life expectancy of > 10 years, and with no significant comorbidity.

3. Advanced disease. This is best treated with hormone manipulation.

4. Hormonal therapy. As most CaP cells are androgen sensitive reducing the level of dihydrotestosterone (DHT) available to these cells can lead to apoptosis (programmed cell death) with resultant reduction in tumour volume and delay in disease progression. This can be achieved by a number of methods:

- Bilateral orchidectomy.
- Non-steroidal anti-androgens (e.g. cyproterone acetate, flutamide, bicalutamide). These block the nuclear receptor for DHT.

- Luteinizing hormone releasing hormone (LHRH) agonists. (e.g. leuprorelin, goserilin).

These drugs, now available in 3-monthly depot injections, desensitize the LHRH receptors in the pituitary, inhibiting luteinizing hormone release and thus testosterone production.

5. Complications of bony metastases

- Pain can be treated with analgesics or with palliative radiotherapy.
- More widespread bony pain can be treated with radioactive isotopes which have a high affinity for the skeleton such as strontium-89.
- Cord compression. This is a catastrophic complication of bony metastases if not recognized early. The level of metastatic compression of the spinal cord can be confirmed by MRI and prompt treatment with radiotherapy may prevent permanent neurological sequelae.

Further reading

Crawford *et al.* Overview: hormone refractory prostatic carcinoma. *Urology*, 1999; **54**: 1–7.
Hegarty *et al.* Future prospects in prostate carcinoma. *Prostate*, 1999; **40**: 261–268.

RADIOLOGICAL INVESTIGATIONS

Pathology arising in the renal tract can be demonstrated by several imaging techniques. Occasionally there is sufficient natural contrast between the pathology, or its effects, and adjacent normal structures for plain X-rays to be sufficient. Alternatively it may be necessary to use contrast agents.

The choice of any radiological investigations should be targeted based on the provisional and differential diagnosis generated by the history and physical examination.

X-ray images

X-rays are examples of electromagnetic waves. Quantum mechanics regards electromagnetic waves as packets of energy (photons) travelling with the velocity of light.

The radiographic image

In generating an X-ray image X-ray photons are projected at the patient. Some of these photons are stopped by the tissues of the body, others are not. Those that get all the way through the patient to emerge from the opposite side and reach the X-ray film are the ones that are responsible for creating the image.

Intravenous pyelogram

An intravenous pyelogram (IVP) is performed by injecting iodinated contrast material into a vein. An IVP is useful in patients with haematuria, hydronephrosis or abdominal pain thought to be related to the kidneys.

An IVP, however, is an invasive test. It requires placement of an intravenous line. Because significant renal function is required to concentrate and excrete the contrast material, IVPs are not useful in patients with renal dysfunction.

A plain X-ray film from the area of the kidneys, ureters and bladder (KUB) is taken first as a control film. A single view plain film may be sufficient to diagnose the presence of a ureteral stone. It is low cost with low radiation exposure and may be done rapidly within the urology clinic. The plain film is limited by its low sensitivity for detection of opaque as well as non-opaque stones. Recent studies have shown a sensitivity of about 50% for stone visualization with the abdominal film. Occasionally a suspected ureteral calcification seen on plain film turns out to be a vascular phlebolith when more specific studies are performed. As the contrast is excreted by the kidney, X-rays are obtained. An IVP is a useful test to determine both anatomy and function. It provides high resolution images so that the renal pelvis, calyces and ureter are all well seen. Absence of function or perfusion to a kidney can be detected when no contrast is excreted.

Newborns rarely have sufficient renal concentrating ability to allow the kidneys to be seen on an X-ray. An IVP will detect renal function, but it is not very sensitive in comparing the function of two kidneys. Nuclear renograms are the best G/U imaging study to measure renal function. If a renal tumour is suspected an ultrasound would be a better study.

Ultrasound

The imaging technique of ultrasound uses, as the name implies, sound waves transmitted through tissue. The prefix 'ultra' indicates that the sound waves in question have a frequency somewhat higher than audible 'sound'. The human ear can detect frequencies ranging from 20 Hz to 20 kHz. The frequencies used in diagnostic ultrasound vary from 1 to 10 MHz. The higher the frequency of the ultrasound wave the less tissue penetration but the greater the resolution of near objects. Abdominal ultrasound imaging of the kidney uses 3.5 MHz and trans-rectal prostate imaging utilizes 7.5 MHz.

Computerized tomography (CT)

Conventional radiographs depict a three-dimensional object as a two-dimensional image. Their main limitation is that overlying tissues are superimposed on the image. Computed tomography overcomes this problem by scanning thin slices of the body with a narrow X-ray beam which rotates around the body, producing an image of each slice as a cross-section of the body and showing each of the tissues in a 10-mm slice. Another limitation of the conventional radiograph is its inability to distinguish between two tissues with similar density, such as soft tissue and fluid. Computed tomography can differentiate between tissues of similar density because of the narrow X-ray beam and the use of 'windowing'.

The information acquired by computed tomography is stored on computer as digital raw data and an image can be displayed on a video monitor or printed on to X-ray film. The image is made up of a matrix of thousands of tiny squares or pixels (65 000 pixels in a conventional image). Each pixel has a computed tomography number (measured in Hounsfield units) attributed to it. The computed tomography number is a measure of how much of the initial X-ray beam is absorbed by the tissues at each point in the body. This varies according to the density of the tissues. The denser the tissue is the higher the computed tomography number, ranging from 1000 HU (air) to 1000 HU (bone).

CT is most important for the evaluation of detecting and staging of solid renal lesions. It is also becoming of great importance for the evaluation of patients with trauma and investigations of stone disease.

Magnetic resonance imaging (MRI)

The patient is put into a large magnetic field. The spinning protons of hydrogen nuclei act as small bar magnets. These align with or against the field. A radiofrequency (RF) pulse of electro-magnetism is then passed across the patient. The bar magnets resonate with the frequency and flip. After the RF pulse has stopped they return to their original alignment with or against the field. As they do so they give out a radio wave. This is picked up by a detector and by complex mathematics turned into a picture based on the frequency, phase and amplitude.

The return to equilibrium is called magnetic relaxation and is a unique property of each tissue described as T1 and T2 relaxation times. These are important determinants of image contrast and signal intensity in MRI.

The benefits of MRI are that there is no ionizing radiation or need for iodinated contrast. The images are three-dimensional giving better soft tissue differentiation and improved imaging of vascular structures.

MRI is useful in evaluating the limits of vena caval involvement in renal carcinoma, evaluation of spinal cord compression in patients with metastatic disease and has some use in staging of localized prostatic carcinoma.

Nuclear medicine

1. Nuclear renogram. A nuclear renogram is performed by injecting a radioisotope into a vein. The isotope flows through the blood vessels of the kidney and is filtered by the glomerulus and/or secreted by the renal tubules. As the isotope flows into the collecting system, it is detected by a nuclear medicine camera usually placed posterior to the kidneys. The amount of isotope filtered and drained by the kidneys can be analysed by a computer. In this way, perfusion, function and drainage of the kidney can all be determined A nuclear renogram is useful when questions arise about obstruction of a kidney (hydronephrosis), compromise of a kidney's blood flow, or relative function of a kidney. Nuclear renograms are very sensitive at detecting renal function. However, they have very low resolution. They are really just a collection of black dots. A nuclear renogram may detect obstruction of a kidney, but the films would not indicate the specific anatomy of the kidney, renal pelvis or ureter. An intravenous pyelogram (IVP) would better show such anatomy in a kidney with relatively good renal function. A nuclear renogram is useful in evaluating hydronephrosis (to determine function of the kidney and to detect obstruction) or abnormal renal parenchyma seen on ultrasound (to evaluate function). Nuclear renograms are very useful in evaluating a kidney transplant (to evaluate function).

Radioisotopic renography is important because it provides information regarding differential renal function and the velocity of emptying of the renal pelvis. Technetium-99m diethylenetriaminepentaacetic acid (DTPA), an agent excreted almost exclusively by filtration, is known to provide accurate information regarding glomerular filtration rate in non-dilated kidneys. The accuracy of such determinations in the presence of hydronephrosis is controversial. Mercaptoacetyltriglycine (MAG3), on the other hand, is excreted mostly by the renal tubules. What is measured by studying the differential uptake of this agent by the kidneys is not clear; however, because it yields better images in infants and patients with compromised renal function, it has become the preferred agent in many centres.

The pattern of the excretory curve of the renogram reflects the speed of emptying of the renal pelvis. Because dilated collecting systems retain the isotope for prolonged periods of time even when not obstructed, frusemide is usually given to promote diuresis and emptying. Although the diuretic renogram can supply very useful information, clinicians should keep in mind that there are several factors which can make the results unreliable. First of all, poor renal function may cause an inability to respond to the diuretic, resulting in a false delay in washout time. Poor hydration may also limit the response to diuretic. Secondly, there is no standard protocol for the administration or the interpretation of the diuretic renogram. Care should be taken when comparing studies performed in two different institutions. It is crucial that a standard protocol be developed and maintained at all times within a single centre to facilitate comparison of scans over time. Finally, the diuretic renogram identifies the presence of obstruction but not the cause of obstruction. There is very little anatomic detail provided with the diuretic renogram.

Bone scans

With the array of methods currently available to evaluate the musculoskeletal system, deciding among plain-film radiography, magnetic resonance imaging

(MRI), computed tomography (CT) and nuclear medicine imaging can be difficult. Bone scintigraphy is not the newest but remains one of the most commonly performed studies in nuclear medicine, because it is useful in several diseases and conditions.

Technetium Tc 99m methylene diphosphonate is the radiopharmaceutical agent most commonly used in bone scintigraphy. The phosphonate compounds bind to bone by chemiadsorption to the hydroxyapatite crystal. Technetium 99m decays by releasing 140-kV gamma rays, which are detected by a gamma camera. The appearance of activity on the scan usually reflects osteoblastic activity in bone.

Images can be obtained immediately after technetium injection; they reflect the initial blood pool and flow and are useful in assessing vascularity. However, for optimal evaluation of bone activity, image acquisition should be delayed for 2–3 h. Occasionally, when initial bladder activity may be a problem in pelvic assessment, image acquisition is delayed for 24 h.

In general, planar images (two-dimensional, analogous to plain films) are used. However, in certain circumstances, single-photon emission computed tomography (SPECT) images are required to increase sensitivity and aid in localization.

Findings indicating malignant versus benign tumour

The most common presentation of widespread metastatic disease is multiple asymmetric foci of abnormally increased activity involving the axial and, to a lesser extent, the appendicular skeleton. These findings are often pathognomonic of metastatic disease. However, most patients with suspected metastasis are older adults and can have active osteoarthritis or other benign diseases that cause increased activity on bone scintigraphy. Although further imaging with plain films, CT or MRI may be needed to clarify findings, certain patterns can often be recognized and interpreted with confidence as benign.

For example, increased activity in the sternoclavicular or sternomanubrial joints or costochondral junctions is usually benign and secondary to degenerative changes. Lesions in two or more adjacent ribs typically suggest benign fractures, whereas an elongated lesion along a rib or asymmetric lesions in the sternum suggest malignant disease.

In the spine, malignant lesions usually involve the vertebral body, possibly extending into the pedicles and rarely into the spinous process. Increased activity in adjacent vertebral end plates, in the posterior neural arch (including the facet joints), or in transverse or spinous processes alone, as well as the presence of lesions extending beyond the normal border of the vertebral body, usually indicates benign or degenerative disease.

Diagnostic radiology during pregnancy

Because of the possibility of fetal malformation, genetic damage or subsequent childhood malignancy, radiation exposure of the lower abdomen and pelvis of pregnant women should be kept to a minimum.

Often, the radiological examination can be postponed until after pregnancy, but if it is considered that the possible benefits outweigh any risks, the radiological examination should be performed with the minimum fetal radiation dose, using the smallest practicable beam size, fastest film-screening combination and as few exposures as practical.

Most diagnostic radiological procedures carried out as planned procedures, or occurring inadvertently when it is not realized that the patient is pregnant, will give a fetal radiation dose of less than 20 mGy (2 rads). In these instances, that patient can be reassured that there is minimal risk of sequelae.

If during pregnancy it is suspected that the fetal radiation dose is greater than 20 MGy (2 rads), the exposure should be accurately estimated by a medical physicist. Such a dose may be received from a sequence of radiological procedures or multiple radiographic exposures and/or prolonged fluoroscopy with the maternal pelvis in the primary beam. Usually the fetal exposure will be found to be less than 100 MGy (10 rads) and the patient can be reassured that the risk is negligible compared with the overall 4% to 6% risk of congenital defects during pregnancy.

In the rare instance when the fetus is thought to have received a radiation dose greater than 100 MGy, the radiation exposure must be accurately estimated by a medical physicist. Subsequent management will depend on a number of factors, including the stage of gestation, the patient's age, and her desire to proceed with the pregnancy. However, as the risk of fetal abnormalities is significantly increased above control levels only at doses about 150 MGy, and as the dose to the fetus will rarely reach or exceed this figure, exposure of the fetus to radiation from diagnostic procedures would only rarely be a cause by itself, for terminating a pregnancy.

RENAL CELL CARCINOMA

Renal cell carcinoma accounts for approximately 3% of adult malignancies and 90–95% of neoplasms arising from the kidney. It is characterized by a lack of early warning signs, diverse clinical manifestations, resistance to radiation and chemotherapy, and infrequent but reproducible responses to immunotherapy agents such as interferon alpha and interleukin (IL)-2. In the past it was believed that these tumours derived from the adrenal gland; therefore, the term hypernephroma often was used.

The tissue of origin for renal cell carcinoma is the proximal renal tubular epithelium. Renal cancer occurs in both a sporadic (non-hereditary) and a hereditary form. Familial and sporadic forms of renal cell carcinoma are associated with structural alterations of the short arm of chromosome 3 (3p). Genetic studies of the families at high risk for developing renal cancer led to the cloning of genes whose alteration results in tumour formation. These genes are either tumour suppressors (*VHL, TSC*) or oncogenes (*MET*).

At least four hereditary syndromes associated with renal cell carcinoma are recognized:

1. Von Hippel–Lindau (VHL) syndrome.
2. Hereditary papillary renal carcinoma (HPRC).
3. Familial renal oncocytoma (FRO) associated with Birt–Hogg–Dube syndrome (BHDS).
4. Hereditary renal carcinoma (HRC).

VHL disease is transmitted in an autosomal dominant familial multiple-cancer syndrome, in which there is predisposition to a variety of neoplasms, including the following:

- Renal cell carcinoma with clear cell histology.
- Phaeochromocytoma
- Pancreatic cysts and islet cell tumours
- Retinal angiomas
- Central nervous system haemangioblastomas
- Endolymphatic sac tumours
- Epididymal cystadenomas.

Renal cell carcinoma develops in nearly 40% of patients with VHL disease and is a major cause of death among these patients. Deletions of 3p occur commonly in renal cell carcinoma associated with VHL disease. The *VHL* gene is mutated in a high percentage of tumours and cell lines from patients with sporadic (non-hereditary) clear cell renal carcinoma. Several kindreds with familial clear cell carcinoma have a constitutional balanced translocation between 3p and either chromosome 6 or chromosome 8.

HPRC is an inherited disorder with an autosomal dominant inheritance pattern in which individuals who are affected develop bilateral, multifocal papillary renal carcinoma. Germline mutations in the tyrosine kinase domain of the *MET* gene have been found recently.

In FRO, individuals can develop bilateral, multifocal oncocytoma or oncocytic neoplasms in the kidney. BHDS is a hereditary cutaneous syndrome. Patients with this syndrome have a dominantly inherited predisposition to develop benign tumours of the hair follicle (fibrofolliculomas), predominantly on the face, neck, and upper trunk and are at risk of developing renal tumours, colon polyps or tumours, and pulmonary cysts.

Mortality/morbidity

Renal cell carcinoma is the sixth leading cause of cancer death. The 5-year survival rates initially reported by Robson in 1969 were 66% for stage I renal carcinoma, 64% for stage II, 42% for stage III, and only 11% for stage IV. Except for stage I, these survival statistics have remained essentially unchanged for several decades.

Race

Renal cell carcinoma is more common in people of Northern European ancestry (Scandinavians) and North Americans than in those of Asian or African descent.

Sex

Renal cell carcinoma is twice as common in men as in women.

Age

This condition occurs most commonly in the fourth to sixth decades of life, but the disease has been reported in family clustering at a younger age.

Presentation

Renal cell carcinoma may remain clinically occult for most of its course. The classic triad of flank pain, haematuria and flank mass is infrequent (10%) and is indicative of advanced disease. Twenty-five to 30% of patients are asymptomatic, and renal cell carcinoma is found on incidental radiologic study.

- Most common presentations
  - (i) Haematuria (40%)
  - (ii) Flank pain (40%)
  - (iii) Palpable mass in the flank or abdomen (25%)
- Other signs and symptoms
  - (i) Weight loss (33%)
  - (ii) Fever (20%)
  - (iii) Hypertension (20%)
  - (iv) Hypercalcaemia (5%)
  - (v) Night sweats
  - (vi) Malaise
  - (vii) Varicocele, usually left sided, due to obstruction of the testicular vein (2% of males)
- Renal cell carcinoma is a unique and challenging tumour because of the frequent occurrence of paraneoplastic syndromes, including hypercalcaemia, erythrocytosis, and non-metastatic hepatic dysfunction (Stauffer syndrome). Polyneuromyopathy, amyloidosis, anaemia, fever, cachexia, weight loss, dermatomyositis, increased sedimentation rate and hypertension also are associated with renal cell carcinoma.
  - (i) Cytokine release by tumour (e.g. IL-6, erythropoietin, nitric oxide) causes these paraneoplastic findings.
  - (ii) Resolution of symptoms or biochemical abnormalities frequently follows successful treatment of the primary tumour or metastatic foci.

Examination

- Gross haematuria with vermiform clots suggests upper urinary tract bleeding.
- Hypertension, supraclavicular adenopathy, and flank or abdominal mass with bruit.
- Approximately 30% of patients with renal carcinoma present with metastatic disease. Physical examination should include thorough evaluation for metastatic disease. Organs involved include:
  (i)   Lung (75%)
  (ii) Soft tissues (36%)
  (iii) Bone (20%)
  (iv) Liver (18%)
  (v)   Cutaneous sites (8%)
  (vi) Central nervous system (8%)
- Varicocele and findings of paraneoplastic syndrome raise clinical suspicion for this diagnosis.

Investigations

- Laboratory studies in the evaluation of renal cell carcinoma should include a workup for paraneoplastic syndromes. Initial studies are as follows:
  (i)   Urine analysis
  (ii) Full blood count with differential count
  (iii) Electrolytes
- Liver function test
- Calcium
- Erythrocyte sedimentation rate
- Prothrombin time
- Activated partial thromboplastin time.

Radiological investigations

A large proportion of patients diagnosed with renal cancer have small tumours discovered incidentally on imaging studies. A number of diagnostic modalities are used to evaluate and stage renal masses, including the following:

- Excretory urography
- Computed tomography scan
- Ultrasonography
- Arteriography
- Venography
- Magnetic resonance imaging

1. Determining whether a space-occupying renal mass is benign or malignant can be difficult. Radiological studies should be tailored to enable further characterization of renal masses, so that non-malignant tumours can be differentiated from malignant ones.
2. Excretory urography is not frequently used in the initial evaluation of renal masses because of its low sensitivity and specificity. A small-to-medium-sized tumour may be missed by excretory urography.

3. Contrast-enhanced CT scanning has become the imaging procedure of choice for diagnosis and staging of renal cell cancer and has virtually replaced excretory urography and renal ultrasound. In most cases, CT imaging can differentiate cystic masses from solid masses and supplies information about lymph nodes and renal vein and inferior vena cava involvement.
4. Ultrasound examination provides excellent staging and diagnostic information. Ultrasound provides accurate anatomic detail of extra-renal extension of tumour, adrenal or lymph node involvement, and infiltration of adjacent viscera. Ultrasonography can be useful in evaluating questionable cystic renal lesions if CT imaging is inconclusive. Large papillary renal tumours are frequently undetectable by renal ultrasound.
5. Renal arteriography is not used in the evaluation of suspected renal mass as frequently now as it was in the past. When inferior vena cava involvement is suspected, either inferior venacavography or MRI is used. MRI is currently the preferred imaging technique. Inferior vena cava involvement is important in planning the vascular aspect of the operative procedure.
6. A bone scan is recommended for bony symptoms with elevated alkaline phosphatase.

Histologic findings

Renal cell carcinoma has five histological subtypes, as follows: clear cell (75%), chromophilic (15%), chromophobe (5%), oncocytoma (3%), and collecting duct (2%). Unusually clear cells with a cytoplasm rich in lipids and glycogen characterize clear cell carcinoma, which is most likely to show 3p deletion.

Chromophilic tumours tend to be bilateral and multifocal and may have trisomy 7 and/or trisomy 17.

Large polygonal cells with pale reticular cytoplasm characterize chromophobe carcinoma and do not exhibit 3p deletion.

Renal oncocytoma consists predominantly of eosinophilic cells, in a characteristic nested or organoid pattern, that rarely metastasize and do not exhibit 3p deletion or trisomy 7 or 17.

Collecting duct carcinoma is an unusual variant characterized by a very aggressive clinical course. This tends to affect younger patients and may present with local or widespread advanced disease. These cells can have three different types of growth patterns: (1) acinar, (2) sarcomatoid, and (3) tubulopapillary. The sarcomatoid variant, which can occur with any histologic cell type, is associated with a significantly poorer prognosis.

Staging

- The Robson modification of the Flocks and Kadesky system is uncomplicated and commonly used in clinical practice. This system was employed to correlate stage at presentation with prognosis. The Robson staging system is as follows:
  (i)   Stage I – Tumour confined within capsule of kidney.
  (ii) Stage II – Tumour invading perinephric fat but still contained within the Gerota fascia.

(iii) Stage III – Tumour invading the renal vein or inferior vena cava (A), or regional lymph-node involvement (B), or both (C).

(iv) Stage IV – Tumour invading adjacent viscera (excluding ipsilateral adrenal) or distant metastases.

- The tumour, nodes and metastases (TNM) classification is endorsed by the American Joint Committee on Cancer (AJCC). The major advantage of the TNM system is that it clearly differentiates individuals with tumour thrombi from those with local nodal disease. In the Robson system, stage III inferior vena caval involvement (IIIA) is the same stage as local lymph node metastases (IIIB). Although patients with Robson stage IIIB renal carcinoma have greatly decreased survival rates, the prognosis for patients with Robson stage IIIA renal carcinoma is not markedly different from that for patients with Robson stage I or II renal carcinoma. The TNM classification system is as follows:

(i) Primary tumour (T)
- TX – Primary tumour cannot be assessed
- T0 – No evidence of primary tumour
- T1 – Tumour 7 cm or smaller in greatest dimension, limited to the kidney
- T2 – Tumour larger than 7 cm in greatest dimension, limited to the kidney
- T3 – Tumour extends into major veins or invades adrenal gland or perinephric tissues but not beyond the Gerota fascia.
- T3a – Tumour invades adrenal gland or perinephric tissues but not beyond the Gerota fascia.
- T3b – Tumour grossly extends into the renal vein(s) or vena cava below the diaphragm.
- T3c – Tumour grossly extends into the renal vein(s) or vena cava above the diaphragm.
- T4 – Tumour invading beyond the Gerota fascia.

(ii) Regional lymph nodes (N) (laterality does not affect the N classification)
- NX – Regional lymph nodes cannot be assessed.
- N0 – No regional lymph node metastasis.
- N1 – Metastasis in a single regional lymph node.
- N2 – Metastasis in more than 1 regional lymph node.

(iii) Distant metastasis (M)
- MX – Distant metastasis cannot be assessed.
- M0 – No distant metastasis.
- M1 – Distant metastasis.

(iv) AJCC stage I – T1, N0, M0.

(v) AJCC stage II – T2, N0, M0.

(vi) AJCC stage III – T1–2, N1, M0 or T3a–c, N0–1, M0.

(vii) AJCC stage IV – T4; or any T, N2, M0; or any T, any N, M1.

Surgical care

Surgical resection remains the only known effective treatment for localized renal cell carcinoma, and it also is used for palliation in metastatic disease.

Radical nephrectomy, which is the standard procedure today for treatment of localized renal carcinoma, involves complete removal of Gerota's fascia and its contents, including a resection of kidney, perirenal fat and ipsilateral adrenal gland, with or without ipsilateral lymph node dissection. Radical nephrectomy provides a better surgical margin than simple removal of the kidney, since perinephric fat may be involved in some patients. Twenty to 30% of patients with clinically localized disease develop metastatic disease after nephrectomy. Some surgeons believe that the adrenal gland should not be removed, due to low probability of ipsilateral adrenal metastasis and morbidity associated with adrenalectomy. In the absence of distant metastatic disease with locally extensive and invasive tumours, adjacent structures such as bowel, spleen or psoas muscle may be excised en bloc during radical nephrectomy.

Lymph nodes may be involved in 10–25% of patients. The 5-year survival rate in patients with regional node involvement is substantially lower than in patients with stage I and II disease. Regional lymphadenectomy adds little in terms of operative time or risk and should be included in conjunction with radical nephrectomy.

Approximately 5% of patients with renal cell carcinoma have inferior vena caval involvement. Tumour invasion of the renal vein and inferior vena cava usually occurs as a well-vascularized thrombus covered with its own intimal surface. In patients with renal vein involvement without metastases, radical nephrectomy is performed with early ligation of the renal artery but no manipulation of the renal vein. If the inferior vena cava is involved, then vascular control of the inferior vena cava is obtained both above and below the tumour thrombus, and the thrombus is resected intact, with subsequent closure of the vena cava. Patients with actual invasion of the inferior vena caval wall have poor prognoses, despite aggressive surgical approaches.

At least three common approaches exist for removal of kidney cancer, as follows:

1. Transperitoneal approach.
2. Flank approach.
3. Thoracoabdominal approach.

The approach depends on the location and tumour size and the body habitus of the patient. The thoracoabdominal approach offers the advantage of palpation of the ipsilateral lung cavity and mediastinum, as well as the ability to resect solitary pulmonary metastases.

Laparoscopic nephrectomy is a less invasive procedure. Laparoscopic surgery tends to incur less morbidity and is associated with shorter recovery time and less blood loss. The need for pain medications is reduced, but operating room time and costs are higher. Disadvantages include concerns about spillage, limited experience and technical difficulties in defining surgical margins. Laparoscopic nephrectomy is an attractive alternative to the removal of kidneys with a small-volume renal cell cancer.

Palliative nephrectomy is considered in patients with metastatic disease for alleviation of symptoms such as pain, haemorrhage, malaise, hypercalcaemia, erythrocytosis or hypertension. Reports have documented regression of metastatic renal cell carcinoma after removal of the primary tumour. Adjuvant nephrectomy is not recommended for inducing spontaneous regression; rather, it is performed to decrease symptoms or to decrease tumour burden for subsequent therapy in carefully controlled environments.

About 25–30% of patients have metastatic disease at diagnosis, and fewer than 5% have solitary metastasis. Surgical resection is recommended in selected patients with metastatic renal carcinoma. This procedure may not be curative in all patients but may produce some long-term survivors. The possibility of disease-free survival increases after resection of primary tumour and isolated metastasis excision.

Medical care

More than 50% of patients with renal cell carcinoma are cured in early stages, but outcome for stage IV disease is poor. The probability of cure is directly related to the stage or degree of tumour dissemination, so the approach is curative for early stage disease. Selected patients with metastatic disease respond to immunotherapy, but many patients can be offered only palliative therapy for advanced disease. The treatment options for renal cell cancer are surgery, radiation therapy, chemotherapy, hormonal therapy, immunotherapy or combinations of these.

Options for systemic therapy are limited, and no hormonal or chemotherapeutic regimen is accepted as a standard of care. Objective response rates, either for single or combination chemotherapy, usually are lower than 15%. Therefore, various biologic therapies have been evaluated.

Renal cell carcinoma is an immunogenic tumour, and spontaneous regressions have been documented. Many immune modulators, such as interferon, IL-2 (aldesleukin or proleukin), bacillus Calmette-Guérin (BCG) vaccination, lymphokine-activated killer (LAK) cells plus IL-2, tumour-infiltrating lymphocytes, and non-myeloablative allogeneic peripheral blood stem-cell transplantation have been tried.

Follow-up

For stage I and II disease, complete history, physical examination, chest X-ray, liver function test, urea and creatinine, and calcium are recommended every 6 months for 2 years, then annually for 5 years. Abdominal CT scan is recommended once at 4–6 months and then as indicated.

For stage III renal cell carcinoma, physical examination, chest X-ray, liver function tests, urea N and creatinine, and calcium are recommended every 4 months for 2 years, every 6 months for 3 years, and then annually for 5 years. Abdominal CT scan should be performed at 4–6 months, then annually or as indicated.

Spontaneous regression has been reported anecdotally in renal cell carcinoma. Up to 10% of patients with metastatic disease show no progression for more than 12 months. All systemic therapies are associated with treatment-related toxicity and low response, so close observation is an option for asymptomatic metastatic disease. Once evidence of progression or symptoms occurs, appropriate therapy should be initiated.

Careful surveillance of patients with end-stage renal disease using ultrasonography and CT scan is recommended.

Prognosis

Metastatic disease has increased survival with (1) a long disease-free interval between initial nephrectomy and the appearance of metastases, (2) the presence of only pulmonary metastases, (3) good performance status, and (4) removal of the primary tumour.

1. *Five-year survival rates.* After radical nephrectomy for stage I renal cell carcinoma, the 5-year survival rate is approximately 94%, and patients with stage II lesions have a survival rate of 79%. A tumour confined to the kidney is associated with a better prognosis.

The 5-year disease-specific survival rate of T1 renal carcinoma is 95% and is 88% with stage T2 disease. Patients with T3 renal carcinoma had a 59% 5-year survival rate, and those with T4 disease had a 20% 5-year disease-specific survival rate.

Patients with regional lymph node involvement or extracapsular extension have a survival rate of 12–25%. Although renal vein involvement does not have a markedly negative effect on prognosis, the 5-year survival rate for patients with stage IIIB renal cell carcinoma is 18%. In patients with effective surgical removal of the renal vein or inferior vena caval thrombus, the 5-year survival rate is 25–50%.

Five-year survival rates for patients with stage IV disease are low (0–20%). In a recent trial, five prognostic factors for predicting survival in patients with metastatic renal cell carcinoma were identified. These factors are used to categorize patients with metastatic renal cell carcinoma into three risk groups. Patients in the favourable-risk group (zero risk factors) had a median survival of 20 months. Patients with intermediate risk (1 or 2 risk factors) had a median survival of 10 months, while patients in the poor-risk group (3 or more risk factors) had a median survival of only 4 months. The prognostic factors were as follows:

- Low Karnofsky performance status (<80%).
- High serum lactate dehydrogenase (>1.5 times upper limit of normal).
- Low haemoglobin (below lower limit of normal).
- High 'corrected' serum calcium (>10 mg/dl).
- Absence of prior nephrectomy.

RENAL CYSTIC DISEASE

Recessive polycystic kidney disease (RPKD)

This condition is inherited in an autosomal recessive pattern, giving a 25% recurrence risk for parents having subsequent children. The kidneys are affected bilaterally, so that in utero, there is typically oligohydramnios because of poor renal function and failure to form significant amounts of fetal urine. The most significant result from oligohydramnios is pulmonary hypoplasia, so that newborns do not have sufficient lung capacity to survive, irrespective of any attempt to treat renal failure. RPKD may be termed 'Type I' cystic disease in the Potter's classification.

Grossly, the kidneys are markedly enlarged and tend to fill the retroperitoneum and displace abdominal contents. The kidneys tend to be symmetrically enlarged. The cysts are quite small and uniform, perhaps 1 to 2mm on average. Microscopically, the characteristic finding in the later third trimester is cystic change with the cysts elongated and radially arranged. The few remaining glomeruli are not involved by the cysts, and the intervening parenchyma is not increased. In the second trimester, the cysts may not be as well-developed. A helpful finding at autopsy is the presence of congenital hepatic fibrosis, which accompanies RPKD.

Multicystic renal dysplasia

This condition has a sporadic inheritance pattern. It is perhaps the most common form of inherited cystic renal disease. It results from abnormal differentiation of the metanephric parenchyma during embryologic development of the kidney. However, in many cases it can be unilateral, so the affected person survives, because one kidney is more than sufficient to sustain life. In fact, with absence of one functional kidney from birth, the other kidney undergoes compensatory hyperplasia and may reach a size similar to the combined weight of two kidneys (400 to 500g).

Multicystic renal dysplasia was termed 'Type II' in the Potter classification. There are two main subgroups. If the affected kidney is large, then it is termed 'Type IIa'. If the affected kidney is quite small, it can be termed 'hypodysplasia' or 'Type IIb'. Different combinations are possible, so that only one kidney or part of one kidney can be affected and be either larger or small; both affected kidneys can be large or both can be small, or one can be larger and the other small. It is quite common for asymmetry to be present.

Grossly, the cysts are variably sized, from 1mm to 1cm in size, and filled with clear fluid. There are few recognizable glomeruli and tubules microscopically, and the remaining glomeruli are not affected by the cystic change. The hallmark of renal dysplasia is the presence of 'primitive ducts' lined by cuboidal to columnar epithelium and surrounded by a collagenous stroma. This increased stroma may contain small islands of cartilage. The liver will not show congenital hepatic fibrosis.

Multicystic renal dysplasia is often the only finding, but it may occur in combination with other anomalies and be part of a syndrome (e.g. Meckel–Gruber syndrome), in which case the recurrence risk will be defined by the syndrome. If this disease is bilateral, the problems associated with oligohydramnios are present, with pulmonary hypoplasia the rate limiting step for survival.

Dominant polycystic kidney disease (DPKD)

This condition is inherited in an autosomal dominant pattern, so the recurrence risk in affected families is 50%. However, this disease rarely manifests itself before middle age. It may begin in middle-aged to older adults to cause progressive renal failure as the cysts become larger and the functioning renal parenchyma smaller in volume. This is the 'Type III' cystic disease in the Potter classification, but it is rarely manifested prenatally or in children.

Grossly, DPKD results in very large kidneys, perhaps up to 3 or 4 kg or more. The affected kidneys are just a mass of large fluid-filled cysts. There is often haemorrhage into the cysts, so that some can be filled with grumous brown organizing haemorrhage. There may be intervening normal renal parenchyma earlier in the disease, or just fibrotic stroma late in the course. If DPKD is manifested in fetuses and infants, the cysts may involve the glomeruli (so-called 'glomerular cysts'). In adults, it is common for all or part of the liver to also demonstrate polycystic disease, and it is possible in some cases for the liver to be more severely affected, so that hepatic failure results. Patients with DPKD are also prone to have berry aneurysms of the cerebral arteries.

Cystic change with obstruction

In the fetus and newborn with urinary tract obstruction, it is possible for cystic change to occur in the kidneys, in addition to hydroureter, hydronephrosis and bladder dilatation. Depending upon the point of obstruction, either or both kidneys may be involved. For example, posterior urethral valves in a male fetus, or urethral atresia in a male or female fetus, will cause bladder outlet obstruction so that both kidneys are involved. With bladder outlet obstruction, there will be oligohydramnios and the appearance of pulmonary hypoplasia.

Grossly, this form of cystic disease may not be apparent. The cysts may be no more than 1 mm in size. Microscopically, the cysts form in association with the more sensitive developing glomeruli in the nephrogenic zone so that the cysts tend to be in a cortical location. Thus, 'cortical microcysts' are the hallmark of this form of cystic disease, which is 'Type IV' in the Potter's classification. There are no accompanying cystic changes in other organs in association with this disease. However, if the obstruction is at the bladder outlet, oligohydramnios with pulmonary hypoplasia can result.

Miscellaneous cystic renal changes in adults

Perhaps the most common cystic change of all is the appearance of one or more simple renal cysts in adults. These cysts may be only a few millimetres in size, or may reach 10 cm or more. They are rarely numerous enough so that intervening normal parenchyma is not recognizable, and they are very unlikely to be the cause for renal failure. These cysts are lined by a flattened cuboidal epithelium and filled with clear fluid. On occasion, there may be haemorrhage into a larger cyst, and it may appear as a mass lesion that can be difficult to differentiate from a renal cell carcinoma (which may undergo necrosis with haemorrhage). However, the finding of clear cells in the cyst fluid is consistent with renal cell carcinoma.

Persons with renal failure who are on long-term dialysis may develop cystic changes in the kidneys. These cysts may be numerous, but never as large as with

DPKD, and the kidneys are still generally small, because most diseases leading to renal failure produce small, shrunken kidneys with end-stage renal disease.

Clinical findings

1. Symptoms. Pain tends to be the predominant feature and will result from the size of the kidneys and/or infection, obstruction and haemorrhage into a cyst.

2. Signs. Tenderness may be found over one or both renal angles. A palpable mass may also be present. Hypertension has been reported in up to 60% of patients with polycystic kidney disease.

3. Investigations. Ultrasonography is excellent in differentiating between solid and cystic lesions. It is far superior than excretory urography and isotope scanning. CT scanning is also an excellent method to establish the diagnosis.

4. Treatments. Treatments are usually conservative and supportive. Patients should keep well hydrated and placed on a low protein diet. Uraemia and hypertension should be controlled. There is no evidence that removing cysts improves renal function but aspiration or removal of cysts causing pelvic/ureteric obstruction may be indicated.

Further reading

Pirson Y. Autosomal dominant polycystic kidney disease. *European Urology Update Series*, 1996; **5**: 20–24.

RENAL STONES

Classification
- Calyceal
- Staghorn (complete, partial or complex)
- Renal pelvic

Treatment options

*1. **Extracorporeal lithotripsy.*** Indications are:

- Symptomatic calyceal calculi less than 1 cm.
- Renal pelvic calculi (<2 cm).
- Partial staghorn calculi.

A recent study has suggested no significant difference in adverse event rate untreated small asymptomatic lower caliceal calculi. Anatomical variations around the lower pole – namely length, width and the angle between renal pelvis and the lower calyceal infundibulum – can lead to considerable variations in success rates (long narrow infundibulae with an acute angle between the infundibulum and the upper ureter fare worst). Stones >2 cm are usually best treated with an indwelling stent to avoid ureteric obstruction and Steinstrasse formation.

*2. **Retrograde ureteroscopy.*** Indications are:

- Partial staghorn.
- Small renal pelvic stone.
- eswl resistant caliceal calculi.

With the advent of the flexible ureteroscope the whole of the renal collecting system is accessible from below. Renal calculi at any site can be treated this way. The main limitations of this approach are technological. The flexible ureteroscope working channel is small (3 Fr maximum) and the instrument delicate. All instruments passed down the channel must also be flexible so either EHL or laser must be available. Passing any instrument down the working channel stiffens the scope and lessens deflection, making the lower calyx difficult to access if it is very dependent (i.e. same limitations in this area as eswl). Even with the holmium laser fragmentation of large stones can be tedious and the benefits of a less invasive but protracted (and probably multiple) procedure have to be weighed against a more invasive but effective technique such as PCNL.

Percutaneous surgery

*1. **Percutaneous nephrolithotomy (PCNL).*** This was first described by Fernstrom and Johansson in the mid 1970s. Indications are:

- Staghorn calculi.
- Large renal calculi (i.e. >2 cm).
- Calculi resistant to eswl.
- Cysteine stones.

- Distil obstruction (e.g. PUJ obstruction) which can be corrected at the time of PCNL.
- Abnormal body habitus making eswl an impractical proposition.

The procedure is as follows:

- Cystoscopy and catheterization of the relevant ureter (either with a purpose designed balloon occlusion catheter or with a standard ureteric catheter).
- The patient is then rolled prone with pillows supporting hips, chest and ankles (the anaesthetist must take care to avoid any orbital pressure).
- The patient is then rolled prone and contrast introduced through the ureteric catheter.
- This allows puncture of the optimal calyx to access the stone.
- Under fluoroscopic control the collecting system is accessed with a hollow needle of sufficient calibre to allow the passage of a guidewire. The wire is then manipulated within the collecting system (optimally down the ureter).
- The track is dilated to 30 Fr using either a balloon system or fascial dilators in a Seldinger type technique.
- A working sheath is sited to allow nephroscopy.
- The stone is then either fragmented using usually the ultrasonic lithotriptor or removed whole dependent on size.
- At the end of the procedure a tube is left in the kidney (nephrostomy) ensure adequate renal drainage.
- Post-operative plain films assess any residual stones.
- When the urine is clear the urethral catheter is removed.
- A nephrostogram (contrast study) is performed and if free ureteric drainage occurs the tube is removed.

Residual stone can be cleared with eswl or with further PCNL or the combination of both modalities (so-called sandwich therapy). Stone free rates exceed 90% with this combination. Recent publications have addressed the issue of the tubeless PCNL where a ureteric stent is sited at the end of the procedure, this results in less post-operative pain but is only suitable for smaller stones. A number of authors have proposed the mini PCNL where the track is only dilated to 16 or 18 Fr and a paediatric scope is used. This may well prove to be the answer for relatively small lower calyceal calculi which are resistant to eswl and inaccessible to the flexible ureteroscope, but certainly at this time there does not appear to be a significant advantage over standard PCNL.

2. Laparoscopy. In a number of centres laparoscopic pyelolithotomy and more recently anatrophic nephrolithotomy have been reported; as yet the role of laparoscopy is not defined.

- Open surgery. Scalpel surgery is rare in the 21st century with most specialized centres performing <5% of their stone extraction through standard incisional surgery.
- Indications:
  (i) Complex stone burden.
  (ii) Anatomical abnormality (e.g. PUJ obstruction).
  (ii) Failed minimally invasive therapy.

- Pyelolithotomy
  (i) The kidney is exposed via a loin incision and the renal pelvis exposed.
  (ii) The renal pelvis is incised and the stone removed.
  (iii) Various angles of stone forcep are then used to remove any caliceal fragments and the renal pelvis washed out.
  (iv) The renal pelvis is closed over a stent using absorbable sutures and a drain left in the retroperitoneal space.
- Anatrophic nephrolithotomy
  (i) The kidney is exposed as in pyelolithotomy.
  (ii) The kidney is cooled to 20°C using ice slush and the renal vessels clamped.
  (iii) The kidney is incised on the posterior border of its convex surface (the anterior and posterior branches of the renal artery leave a relatively bloodless plane here).
  (iv) Calculi are removed as previously.
  (v) The collecting system and kidney are then closed with absorbable sutures over a nephrostomy catheter.
  (vi) The renal circulation is then restored.
- Radial nephrotomy
  (i) A stab incision is made over the stone.
  (ii) The collecting system is repaired and the kidney closed with absorbable sutures.
  (iii) This is useful combined with pyelolithotomy or when a stone is present in a dilated calyx and can be combined with remodelling of a stenosed infundibulum.

Further reading

Pak C. Kidney stones. *Lancet*, 1998; **351**: 1797–1800.
Segura J *et al.* Nephrolithiasis clinical guidelines panel summary report on the management of staghorn calculi. *Journal of Urology*, 1994; **151**; 1648–1651.
www.duj.com Ramakumar S, Segura JW. Percutaneous management of urinary calculi.

RENAL TRANSPLANTATION

Transplantation of tissues and whole organs has become commonplace. Transplantation is useful for treating a variety of disease conditions not amenable to other therapies. The technical aspects of tissue and organ harvesting are well understood, and the surgical procedures for grafting tissues and organs into the body are also well-documented and reliable. The major problems that limit the usefulness of transplantation include the shortages of available tissues, immunologic rejection phenomena and long-term complications.

The first kidney transplant operations were performed in the 1950s. Kidney transplant operations have been available under the UK National Health Service since the mid-1960s. Since that time approximately 32 500 transplants have taken place. Some 1354 kidney transplants took place in the UK in 1999. At the end of that year nearly 6000 patients were still awaiting a transplant.

Types of transplantation

Transplantation can be categorized by the source of the tissues and organs obtained.

1. Autogenous grafts. These are tissues taken from one part of the body and placed in another part in the same person. Since the tissues come from the same person, there is no problem with rejection. Examples include: autogenous coronary artery bypass grafting, bone marrow, skin and hair.

2. Allografts. These are tissues and organs taken from one person and grafted into another person (within the human species). The grafts may come from donors who are living and related, living but unrelated, or from cadavers. The only situation in which complete immune tolerance can be achieved is with grafts between identical twins. For all other persons, the immunologic differences present potential problems with rejection. However some grafts present little threat of immunologic rejection. These situations arise when the tissues are relatively acellular and express antigens minimally, if at all. Use of these tissues requires no special matching procedures. Such tissues include cornea, bone, heart valves.

3. Xenografts. Tissues can be transplanted from other species, but there are major problems with immunologic incompatibility. Experimental procedures have employed primates and pigs. It is theoretically possible to breed animals that have a genetic constitution that makes their tissues more compatible with humans. One situation in which a xenograft is commonly employed is the use of a porcine heart valve to replace a failing human heart valve. The porcine valve is treated to make it immunologically inert and mechanically stable, and it functions well.

4. Foetal tissue grafts. Foetal tissues have a distinct advantage in transplantation because they are immunologically immature, not having reached a state where they recognize other tissues as 'foreign'. Thus, they offer the potential for providing a graft without the need to worry about immunologic rejection. A problem with this type of transplantation centres on ethical dilemmas in obtaining and using such tissues.

Immunology of renal transplantation

Human tissues express antigens. These antigens are on their surfaces and within them. The most important of these in transplantation are the antigens associated with the major histocompatibility complex (MHC). These are best known as HLA antigens because they were first described on white blood cells (human leukocyte antigens). The genes for the MHC reside on the short arm of chromosome 6 in humans. Each person inherits one gene from each parent to determine the pairs of loci that are present. The purpose of the antigens coded by the genes of the MHC is to bind peptide fragments of foreign proteins (such as proteins from infectious agents) to present to antigen-specific T-lymphocytes. There are three major gene products of the MHC:

1. *Class I antigens.* These are antigens expressed on all nucleated cells and on circulating platelets. The loci are designated as HLA-A, HLA-B, and HLA-C. The antigens bind peptides within cells (typically from viruses that proliferate intracellularly) that are presented to cytotoxic CD8-lymphocytes.

2. *Class II antigens.* These antigens have a limited distribution and are seen mainly on B-lymphocytes, activated T-lymphocytes, monocytes, macrophages, endothelial cells, Langerhans cells, renal epithelial cells and pancreatic beta cells. The loci are designated DR, DP and DQ. They bind peptides that are derived from exogenous antigens (such as from extracellular bacterial infections) and present them to CD4-lymphocytes.

3. *Class III components.* These are the complement components that circulate in the bloodstream.

Transplant rejection can involve both class I and class II HLA antigens. Transplanted tissues that express HLA class I antigens can elicit a cytotoxic CD8-cell response in which there is a hypersensitivity reaction (type II) with direct cytolysis of the cells of the graft. Those tissues expressing HLA class II antigens can provoke a CD4-cell response in which there is a delayed (type IV) hypersensitivity reaction with cytokine activation of macrophages that attack the graft. These two forms of rejection are 'cell-mediated'. In addition, rejection can also occur when B-cells produce circulating antibodies that attack the graft (type III hypersensitivity, antibody-mediated).

Rejection

Hyperacute rejection: this rare complication occurs when there are preformed circulating antibodies in the recipient that immediately attack the engrafted kidney. The kidney ceases functioning within minutes. The immunologic lesion is an Arthus reaction with antigen–antibody complexes deposited in vascular walls, complement activation and neutrophilic infiltration. The extensive vascular injury leads to severe ischaemic injury.

Acute rejection can occur within days or happen months or years following transplantation. Acute rejection takes two forms:

1. *Acute cellular rejection.* Both CD4 and CD8-cells play a role. There is mainly lymphocytic infiltration in a tubulointerstitial distribution.
2. *Acute vascular rejection.* Circulating antibodies deposit in the walls of renal arteries, resulting in a vasculitis, leading to intimal thickening, lumenal narrowing and ischaemia.

Chronic rejection

This may begin to occur months following transplantation. Both cell-mediated and humoral immunologic mechanisms play a role. It is slowly progressive over months. The injury is mainly vascular, with progressive intimal thickening that results in ongoing ischaemia with interstitial fibrosis, tubular atrophy and glomerular sclerosis.

Tissue typing for clinical transplantation

The main purpose of tissue typing in transplantation is (1) to assess donor-recipient compatibility for HLA and ABO blood groups and (2) to analyse patient serum for antibodies that react with transplant donor tissues. Most relevant is the cross-match assay whereby patient sera are tested for their reactivity with donor lymphocytes. This is usually done by lymphocytotoxicity testing whereby donor lymphocytes are first incubated with patient serum, then with rabbit complement and lysis of lymphocytes is assessed by the uptake of an extravital dye like trypan blue or eosin red. A positive cross-match is a contraindication for organ transplantation because of the risk for hyperacute rejection and the higher incidence of vascular rejection during the early post-transplant period.

Transplant candidates may become sensitized following a prior transplant, blood transfusions and previous pregnancies. Serum screening for alloreactive antibodies against a random cell panel will provide an assessment of the degree of sensitization expressed as the percentage Panel Reactive Antibody (PRA). The PRA can vary between 0% (non-sensitized) to 80–100% indicating a high degree of sensitization. Patients with high PRA values are less likely to have cross-match-negative donors. They must wait much longer for a transplant and some may never receive a kidney.

Alloreactive T-lymphocytes are the primary mediators of cellular rejection, and a considerable research effort has emphasized the mixed leukocyte culture (MLC) as an *in vitro* system to determine T-cell alloreactivity between donor and recipient. These MLC assays measure proliferative responses of alloactivated lymphocytes and offer also opportunities to test for cell-mediated cytotoxicity, cytokine production and the quantitation and functional characterization of primed T-cells. Since these MLC procedures are technically demanding and time-consuming, they are not routinely used for prospective histocompatibility testing in a clinical service laboratory.

Considerable evidence has been obtained that matching for HLA will reduce cellular rejection thereby promoting survival of kidney and heart transplant patients. While the HLA system comprises multiple class I and especially class II genes, most matching strategies consider only three loci: HLA-A, HLA-B and HLA-DR. Although it makes sense to find a perfect match for each transplant patient, the reality of clinical practice dictates the selection of less well-matched donors. As noted above, current strategies are directed towards the identification of donors permissible or acceptable HLA mismatches.

Organ retrieval

Guidelines provide information outlining neurological criteria for brain death, which is defined as complete and irreversible loss of brain and brain stem function. Criteria include cerebral unresponsiveness, brainstem areflexia and apnoea in the absence of hypothermia and drug intoxication. The increasing demand for donor organs and improvements in transplant immunology has greatly expanded the pool of patients eligible to donate organs. Absolute contra-indications for transplant donors include HIV, sepsis, and non-CNS malignancy. The task of discussing organ donation with a patient's family is best left to the transplant coordinator, who is highly trained for such discussion.

Following brain death, a number of physiological changes occur, which require intervention to preserve donor organ perfusion. Increasing cerebral oedema after trauma or a cerebral vascular accident initially results in elevated catecholamine release and hypertension. With brain stem necrosis, catecholamine levels drop rapidly to a fraction of normal values, causing hypotension. Such hypotension should be corrected with fluids and vasopressors.

Approximately 75% of organ donors develop diabetes insipidus due to pituitary necrosis. If this condition is untreated, significant hypovolaemia may result. Systemic thermal control often is lost due to hypothalamic ischaemia. This occurs in the majority of donors and results in detrimental effects on potential donor organs, including coagulopathy, hypoxia, hepatic dysfunction and cardiac dysfunction.

Pre-transplant workup summary

1. ABO blood group identical.
2. Least HLA mismatch between donor and recipient with a maximum of three mismatches.
3. Negative cross-match.
4. Recipients aged < 18 years and those with antibodies to HLA tissue types receive priority.
5. When all else is equal, patients who have waited the longest are selected.
6. A full clinical assessment of suitability for transplant is made.

Immunosuppressant treatment

Although individual patients have retained excellent function of their allograft for years without the need for immunosuppression, true tolerance is exceedingly rare, and the majority of patients require long-term immunosuppression. Corticosteroids from the beginning of transplantation have been used for immunosuppression. Their action is to block T-lymphocytes by inhibiting the expression of IL-1 and IL-6.

During the past decade, there has been remarkable progress in our understanding of many of the basic molecular mechanisms of transplant immunology. This has culminated in the release of several new drugs during the past 3 years that have fundamentally altered transplant immunosuppression since cyclosporin A (CsA) was released in 1983.

1. Cyclosporin A. Calcineurin inhibitors remain the cornerstone of successful long-term immunosuppressive regimens. They exert their effects through regulation of cytokine production. CsA was the first agent in this class. CsA significantly reduced rejection rates and improved patient and graft survival in solid organ and bone marrow transplants. It was the first major advance since the synthesis of azathioprine and prednisone in the early 1950s.

Cytokine production is regulated by a series of steps within the T-cells consisting of phosphorylation and dephosphorylation of specific proteins. CsA binds to cyclophilin, a cytosolic protein belonging to the family of immunophilins. This complex can then bind to and inactivate the phosphatase, calcineurin, inhibiting T-cell gene transcription.

2. FK-506 (FK). A second calcineurin inhibitor now available is Tacrolimus or FK-506 (FK). This drug is a macrolide antibiotic isolated from a soil actinomycete. FK was initially approved for use in liver transplantation in 1994. FK has a mechanism of action identical to CsA; however, FK binds to its own unique immunophilin known as 'FK binding protein' (FKBP). The affinity of FK for FKBP is 50 to 100 times greater than that of CsA for its immunophilin. This accounts for the difference in dosage between these agents.

Several large randomized trials comparing CsA with FK in liver and kidney transplantation have been completed. One-year patient and graft-survival rates are not significantly different. However, FK demonstrates superiority in decreasing the rate of acute rejection and in its ability to reverse refractory rejection in the patient treated with CsA.

3. Mycophenolate mofetil. An exciting development concerning inhibitors of RNA and DNA synthesis was the release in 1995 of mycophenolate mofetil (mmF). mmF is a macrolide antibiotic. Its development as a prodrug – the ethyl ester of mycophenolic acid – greatly improves oral bioavailability. mmF selectively inhibits *de novo* purine biosynthesis via inhibition of inosine monophosphate dehydrogenase. This specificity allows for the powerful inhibition of lymphocyte maturation and accounts for the success of mmFs in treating ongoing acute rejection. In a stable patient, the specificity of mmFs eliminates the possibility of toxicity that can result from treatment with the xanthine oxidase inhibitor, allopurinol.

Complications of transplantation

1. Morbidity. Patients who have transplanted organs are at high risk for post-transplant morbidity. Hypertension (46%), cataracts (24%), avascular necrosis (18%), malignant neoplasm (14%), urinary infections (17%), chronic hepatitis (6%), peptic ulcer disease (4%), diverticulitis (3%), myocardial infarction (4%) and cerebrovascular accidents (2%) cause morbidity after renal transplant.

2. Mortality. For all patients receiving long-term dialysis for end-stage renal disease, mortality rates were significantly lower in patients with cadaveric transplants (3.8/100 patients per year) as compared with those persons awaiting transplants (6.3/100 patients per year) and all patients receiving dialysis (16.3/100 patients per year). The greatest increases in life spans were observed in younger patients and in individuals with diabetes.

Recipients of organs from living and related donors have lower mortality rates than recipients of organs from deceased donors. Such patients have fewer episodes of rejection and lower requirements for immunosuppression. Overall, 1-year and 5-year survival rates for such recipients are 99% and 91% respectively. Survival rates for recipients of organs from deceased donors are 95% (1 year) and 81% (5 years).

Graft survival also is related to a living or deceased donor state. If received from a living donor, 1-year and 5-year organ survival rates are 93% and 77% respectively. Graft survival rates from a deceased donor are 87% (1 year) and 62% (5 years).

Causes of mortality in patients with renal transplants vary across different transplant centres. Examples of representative percentages include coronary artery disease (14–50%), sepsis (7–28%), neoplasm (9–28%) and liver failure (0–28%). During the first post-transplant year, most deaths are from infection. Long-term mortality usually is related to coronary artery disease.

Post-transplant complications

1. Infection. Infection is the most common cause of first-year post-transplant mortality and morbidity. Eighty percent of patients with renal transplants experience one or more infections during this period. Infectious agents can often be identified by the time interval from transplant to presentation. The first post-transplant month is dominated by infections directly related to the surgery. The initial 6 months post-transplant are associated with the highest levels of immunosuppression and, thus, have the greatest risk of viral and opportunistic infections. Cytomegalovirus (CMV) is responsible for more than two-thirds of febrile episodes in the first 6 months post-transplant. These patients often present with fever, malaise, lymphadenopathy, arthralgias and myalgias.

After the first 6 months, patients with renal transplants are divided into the following three subgroups: (1) patients with good graft function on minimal immunosuppressants have the same risk of infection as the general population; (2) patients chronically infected with latent viruses (e.g. cmV, EBV, hepatitis B and C) often have significant and ongoing end-organ damage (cirrhosis) due to such infections; and (3) patients with poorly functioning grafts who have sustained multiple episodes of rejection and who require large dosages of immunosuppressants commonly have acute and chronic opportunistic infections.

2. Malignancy. Fifteen years after transplantation, approximately 50% incidence of malignancy exists. The most common sites of cancer are skin (35–40%) followed by viscera (10–15%). Lymphoproliferative malignancies, such as leukaemia and lymphomas, are more prevalent among transplant patients than the general population. Transplant patients are at significantly higher risks for cancers than the general population due to chronic immunosuppression, chronic antigenic stimulation, increased susceptibility to oncogenic viral infections, and direct neoplastic actions of immunosuppressants.

3. Liver disease. Chronic liver disease is an important cause of morbidity and mortality for patients with renal transplants. Aetiologies of hepatic dysfunction include viral hepatitis and anti-rejection therapy. Of the viral infections, cmV is the leading cause of hepatic dysfunction followed by hepatitis C and B. Of anti-rejection medications, azathioprine and cyclosporin are known to cause cholestatic jaundice.

4. Acute renal failure. Failure of renal allografts is now one of the most common causes of end-stage renal disease, accounting for 25% of all patients awaiting renal transplants. Renal transplants can fail for all the same reasons as native kidneys. In addition, renal grafts can fail due to unique causes. Complications of surgery are common causes of graft failure within the first 12 weeks after transplantation. Such complications include renal artery stenosis or thrombosis, urinary tract obstruction and renal vein thrombosis. Recurrent renal disease results in less than 4% of graft failures but may be an important concomitant aetiology of renal failure.

Acute rejection appears within the first 3 months post-transplant and affects 30% of cadaveric and 27% of transplants in living patients. Approximately 20% of patients with transplants will experience recurrent rejection episodes. Patients present with decreasing urine output, hypertension, rising creatinine and mild leukocytosis. Fever, graft swelling, pain and tenderness may be observed with severe rejection episodes. Rejection is secondary to prior sensitization to donor allo-antigens (occult T-cell cross-match) or a positive B-cell cross-match. The final diagnosis depends upon a graft biopsy.

Late-acute rejection is correlated highly with withdrawal of immunosuppressive therapy 6 months after transplantation. Chronic rejection occurs 1 year after transplantation due to immunologic agents and cellular and humoral factors. These patients present with a progressive loss of renal function over time.

5. Cyclosporin toxicity. Cyclosporin and tacrolimus (FK-506) nephrotoxicity are related to haemodynamic factors. Acute cyclosporin toxicity (>300 ng/ml) causes vasoconstriction and renal ischaemia, which can be reversed by decreasing drug dosage. Chronic toxicity results in fixed vascular lesions and irreversible renal ischaemia. Cyclosporin is noteworthy for its many interactions with other medications.

Calcium channel antagonists (e.g. diltiazem, verapamil, nicardipine) and certain antibiotics (e.g. erythromycin, doxycycline, ketoconazole) increase levels of cyclosporin. Certain antibiotics (e.g. nafcillin, co-trimoxazole, isoniazid, rifampin) and certain anticonvulsants (e.g. phenytoin, phenobarbital, carbamazepine) decrease levels of cyclosporin. Drugs that enhance the nephrotoxicity of cyclosporin without altering blood levels include amphotericin B, acyclovir and NSAIDs.

6. Hypertension. Hypertension is found in approximately 50% of all transplant patients. Possible aetiologies of hypertension include graft rejection, cyclosporin toxicity, glomerulonephritis, graft renal artery stenosis, essential hypertension from native kidneys, hypercalcaemia and steroid use.

7. Cardiovascular complications. Overall, risk of cardiovascular disease post transplant is 3–5 times that for age and sex matched controls. Risk factors for such disease include pre-transplant cardiac disease, hyperlipidaemia secondary to anti-rejection medications, hypertension, steroid use, type 1 diabetes mellitus, erythrocytosis, smoking history and multiple previous rejection episodes.

8. Urological complications. Urological complications generally involve leakage and/or obstruction. A 2–10% incidence of ureteral obstruction appears to occur in all renal transplant recipients and obstruction accounts for up to one-third of all significant urological complications. Ureteral obstruction can lead to defunctionalization of the allograft, and is a risk factor for allograft rupture. Recent observations in rodent models of experimental hydronephrosis also demonstrate that pro-inflammatory/pro-fibrogenic cellular and molecular derangements become apparent soon after the onset of obstruction, which could also contribute to allograft failure.

Causes

There are numerous causes of ureteric obstruction including (1) ureteral ischaemia, (2) extrinsic compression-lymphocele, (3) haematoma, (4) abscess, (5) tumour,

(6) ureteral kinking, (7) previously unrecognized ureteropelvic junction obstruction and (8) placement of ureteral anastomosis in mobile anterior dome of bladder. Intrinsic obstruction can be caused by calculi, tumour, clot and oedema.

Obstruction most commonly occurs within 3 months of surgery. The majority of urological complications result from technical error. Diabetes has been shown to contribute to a higher incidence of complications. The use of high doses of corticosteroids, which were administered to patients prior to the advent of cyclosporine, is associated with a higher complication rate, as well as the use of older cadaveric donors.

Most donor ureteral obstructions are distal, and often involve the ureterovesical junction. Distal ischaemia is the most common cause of distal stricture formation. This compromised blood supply can be due to problems in operative technique, or high dose immunosuppression. Upon removal of the donor kidney and ureter, the donor ureter is dependent on the renal artery as its sole source of blood. Two surgical errors may compromise this supply. The first involves stripping the ureter of its adventitia and connective tissue, leading to ischaemia and necrosis of the distal ureter. The second error involves compromise of the ureteral branch of the renal artery by dissecting too high into the renal hilum. Trauma to the renal artery during donor nephrectomy, as caused by excessive traction on the renal vessels during removal, or damage from the perfusion cannula can cause distal ureteral ischaemia.

The technique of ureteral re-implantation into the recipient bladder has been shown to have an impact on the incidence of ureteral obstruction. The techniques generally employed are the Leadbetter–Politano intravesical ureteroneocystostomy, and the Lich extravesical approach. Fewer complications have been reported with the extravesical technique, especially when used with a ureteral stent.

Diagnosis

The diagnosis of ureteral obstruction in a renal transplant recipient is usually made during evaluation of renal failure in an otherwise asymptomatic patient. The denervated graft does not allow the obstruction to cause pain for the recipient. Hydronephrosis may or may not be present. Mild hydronephrosis is quite common in allografts without obstruction. It is generally minimal in early graft obstruction, and is seldom as dramatic in the renal allograft as in the acutely obstructed native kidney. To make matters more confusing, both obstruction and rejection can cause an increased serum creatinine and dilatation in the allograft.

The most definitive diagnostic tool is percutaneous nephrostomy tube placement with antegrade nephrostogram. This method is invasive, but allows visualization and confirmation of stenosis. Allowing the graft to drain via the nephrostomy tube is also therapeutic, and subsequent improvement in function will further confirm the diagnosis.

Retrograde pyelography can also delineate the area of stenosis. However, cannulation of the neo-ureteral orifice may be difficult, and no therapeutic gains are made directly by this procedure. In contrast studies of the transplant ureter, it has been found that mid-ureteral narrowing usually indicates compression, while extensive narrowing along the entire ureteral length usually indicates fibrosis.

Doppler ultrasound and renal scans are used in many centres for the initial diagnostic evaluation of poorly functioning grafts. However, due to minimal dilatation, poor urine output and acute tubular necrosis, these studies may not provide much useful information regarding ureteral obstruction. If renal function is adequate, an intravenous urogram may delineate the obstructed portion of ureter. Ultrasound is the most useful diagnostic tool when lymphocele is suspected as a cause of obstruction. Computerized tomography and magnetic resonance imaging will likely show the cause of obstruction if calculi or extrinsic compression are involved.

Management

After the diagnosis of ureteral obstruction has been made, a variety of therapeutic approaches are available. Prevention, especially in terms of appropriate surgical technique, is very important. As mentioned before, the extravesical ureteroneo-cystostomy has been shown to have a lower incidence of obstruction than the intra-vesical technique. This is especially true when ureteral stenting is employed with the extravesical tecnique. Ureteral stent placement at time of transplantation for select patients has been advocated, mostly for patients with friable bladders, or who have undergone bladder augmentation or urinary diversion. The use of cyclosporine A and the concomitant decrease in corticosteroid dosages also have been beneficial in the prevention of complications.

Management of ureteral obstruction in a renal allograft consists of either endo-urological techniques or open surgery. Because of postoperative peri-ureteral scar-ring, scarring from previous rejection episodes, immunosuppression and renal failure, the endo-urological approach is more desirable when possible. The best candidates for this approach are those with a short stricture in the ureterovesical junction or distal ureter.

Routine ureteral stent placement has been associated with a lower incidence of early postoperative obstruction and subsequent surgery for urological complica-tions. Stents are used to bypass ureteral obstruction. The urine travels primarily between the outside portion of the stent and the ureteral mucosa. Thus, it may become blocked if extrinsic compression is involved.

Further reading

Hodge E. Renal medicine and renal transplantation. *Current Opinions in Urology*, 1997; 101–130.

RENAL TRAUMA

Approximately 10% of all trauma cases involve the genitourinary tract. This is usually blunt trauma and is self-limiting. It has been estimated that 60–90% of all renal injuries occur as a result of blunt trauma but 5–10% of blunt and up to 70% of penetrating trauma are major injuries.

Presentation

The common clinical presentation, which suggests the presence of a renal injury, is evidence of flank trauma (rib fracture/compression injury or bruising), with gross haematuria or with microscopic haematuria with documented evidence of hypotension (systolic blood pressure <90 mmHg). These patients require further radiological/urological investigations. In general patients who present with microscopic haematuria and stable vital signs do not need further urological evaluation. Unstable renal injuries are best treated with prompt surgical exploration. Children under the age of 16 should all undergo radiographic evaluation. Children's kidneys are at higher risk as they are less well protected, more mobile and relatively larger than the adult kidney.

Investigations

Intravenous urogram can be performed after resuscitation has begun and is generally the primary investigation. The urogram should establish the presence or absence of both kidneys, clearly define the renal outlines and cortical borders and outline the collecting systems and ureters.

CT scanning has proved to be an effective means of staging renal trauma and remains the gold standard. It is a non-invasive technique and provides an excellent definition of parenchymal lacerations, clearly defines urinary extravasation and perirenal haematoma. It also gives information on non-viable renal tissue and outlines surrounding organs.

Ultrasonography and renal arteriography may also be used as additional investigations. Arteriography is used when there is a suspicion of venous injury, indeterminate arterial injury on CT scan and patients who may require embolization.

Staging

Staging of renal injuries allows a systematic approach to their management.

1. Radiological staging. Grades 1 and 2 are minor. Grade 1 consists of a contusion or contained subcapsular haematoma without parenchymal laceration. Grade 2; a non-expanding, confined perirenal haematoma or cortical lesion less than 1-cm deep without urinary extravasation. Grades 3, 4 and 5 are major injuries. Grade 3; parenchymal laceration >1 cm without urinary extravasation. Grade 4; parenchymal laceration extending into the collecting system. Grade 5; a shattered kidney with or without damage to the vascular pedicle.

Management

The information from clinical and radiological staging allows for accurate diagnosis.

1. **Blunt injuries.** Minor injuries from blunt trauma account for about 90% of cases and do not require an operation. Bleeding stops spontaneously with bed rest and hydration. The cases which require intervention are those associated with continued retroperitoneal bleeding, urinary extravasation and evidence of non-viable renal parenchyma. Pre-existing renal disease such as hydronephrosis may result in injury to the kidney with more minor trauma.

2. **Penetrating injuries.** Penetrating injuries should be explored. In 80% of penetrating injury, associated organ injury requires operation; thus, renal exploration is only an extension of this procedure. Unfortunately some patients may require emergency laparotomy and renal trauma may have been found unexpectedly. If this occurs an on table IVU is mandatory. If there is extravasation, non-function or calyceal distortion then exploration is indicated. An expanding or pulsatile haematoma also needs exploration but only after vascular control. The midline laparotomy approach is preferred for these injuries. The small bowel needs to be lifted from the abdomen to expose the retroperitoneum. This should be incised just above the origin of the inferior mesenteric artery. Once the left renal vein has been found the left and right renal arteries can be identified. The major vessels can then be secured with tapes. Once vascular control has been established the kidney can be approached by reflecting the colon.

Prognosis

With careful follow-up, most renal injuries have an excellent prognosis, with spontaneous healing and return of renal function. Follow-up blood pressure is vital for the next 3–6 months. An IVU is obtained after 3 months to be certain that perinephric scarring has not caused hydronephrosis or vascular compromise.

Further reading

Nudell *et al.* What to do and when to operate. *Current Opinions in Urology*, 1997; 7: 138–141.

RETROPERITONEAL FIBROSIS

Demography

This condition presents in mid life (40–60 years) and has an incidence of around 1 in 20 000. Males are affected twice as often as females and approximately a third have a non-functioning renal unit at presentation.

Symptoms

Patients present with classical symptoms of back/loin pain radiating anteriorly and into the testicles. The pain is not usually responsive to positional change or opiates though it sometimes responds to aspirin. General malaise, anorexia and occasionally peripheral oedema or symptoms of arterial insufficiency can be present.

Signs

Clinically the stigmata of renal failure may be evident along with hypertension. Peripheral pulses may be diminished and oedema or thrombophlebitis present. In secondary RPF the symptoms of the precipitating condition may be present.

Aetiology and pathology

The majority of cases (60%) are idiopathic Ormond's disease with the remainder secondary to other disease process.

Secondary RPF

Drug therapy	Methysergide (ergot alkaloid)
Malignancy	Colonic, ovarian, breast, lung, lymphoma, cervix, prostate
Pelvic radiotherapy	Ovarian, cervical cancer, seminoma
Aortic aneurysm	Post-repair or inflammatory

Pathologically the aorta, vena cava and ureters are encased in a fibrous plaque centred over the bifurcation of the great vessels which can extend from the level of the renal hilum to the pelvic brim. The middle third of the ureters are drawn medially and encased in the plaque, this holds the ureters rigidly and prevents vermiculation and as such propulsion of the urinary bolus, thus urine drains only by gravity and this results in obstructive renal failure. Occasionally the plaque extends into the mediastinum. The vena cava can occasionally be compromised with resultant peripheral oedema. Rarely the aorta can be compromised with resultant signs and symptoms of arterial insufficiency. Microscopically the plaque contains collagen and fibroblasts with a variable inflammatory infiltrate. Occasionally the ureters or psoas muscle show signs of invasion by the fibrotic process.

Diagnosis and investigation

After full history and clinical examination blood should be taken and analysis of urea and electrolytes, full blood count, ESR and CRP requested. Ultrasound will rapidly allow diagnosis of hydronephrosis, aortic aneurysm and may even identify the fibrotic plaque. IVU characteristically shows hydronephrosis and medial displacement of the middle third of the ureter usually below L3 (IVU is not helpful or safe in the presence of significant renal failure). The best radiological investigation is CT scanning which will readily demonstrate the dilated upper urinary tract and also the fibrotic plaque. Retroperitoneal tumours and lymph nodes will also be noted along with any abnormality of solid visceral organs. Renography is useful to ascertain split function (DMSA, MAG3, DTPA), glomerular filtration rate (Cr EDTA, DTPA) or obstruction (DTPA, MAG3) in the presence of bilateral dilatation on IVU but normal function as judged by serum creatinine. Ultimately the diagnosis of idiopathic fibrosis is on microscopy of biopsy tissue obtained either under radiological control or at the time of laparotomy or laparoscopy.

Management

Initially in the presence of renal failure the kidneys must be decompressed. Ureteric stenting is said to be relatively simple as the ureters are held open (though in the author's experience this is not always so) and can be performed under local or preferably general anaesthesia. If the renal failure is severe and associated with significant fluid overload dialysis may be necessary to optimize the patient's condition. In the presence of sepsis percutaneous nephrostomy is preferable to stenting initially. Retrograde pyelography should precede stent placement and has similar features to IVU. A 6 French stent will usually suffice. In the situation of mild dilatation and normal renal function high-dose steroids have been used (initially 60 mg prednisolone daily) with effect, the disease activity is monitored with serial ESR/CRP estimations and mandatory periodic imaging performed to ensure the hydronephrosis is not progressing. Steroids can be combined with indwelling stents in the frail patient, a reducing course is given but most patients will require maintenance and again regular monitoring of renal function and ESR is mandatory. Surgical management is optimal in the fit patient and involves exposure of the ureters either by medial reflection of the ascending/descending colon or by exposure of the entire retroperitoneum through a posterior peritoneal incision. The ureters are mobilized from the plaque bilaterally and transposed away from the affected area with or without an omental wrap. A biopsy of the plaque is taken. Steroids in a reducing course are usually prescribed and stents left in situ for a short period. Occasionally ureteric resection and re-anastomosis or substitution are necessary. Nephrectomy is indicated in the presence of a non-functioning symptomatic renal unit.

SPINAL INJURIES

It has been stated that 'Among all neurologic disorders, the cost to society of automotive spinal cord injury is exceeded only by the cost of mental retardation'.

Spinal shock is defined as the complete loss of all neurologic function, including reflexes and rectal tone below a specific level associated with autonomic dysfunction. Neurogenic shock refers to the haemodynamic triad of hypotension, bradycardia and peripheral vasodilatation resulting from autonomic dysfunction and the interruption of sympathetic nervous system control in acute spinal cord injury (SCI).

Anatomy

The spinal cord is divided into 31 segments each with a pair of anterior (motor) and dorsal (sensory) spinal nerve roots. On each side, the anterior and dorsal nerve roots combine to form the spinal nerve as it exits from the vertebral column through the neuroforamina. The spinal cord extends from the base of the skull and terminates near the lower margin of the L1 vertebral body. Thereafter, the spinal canal contains the lumbar, sacral and coccygeal spinal nerves comprising the cauda equina.

Injuries below L1, therefore, do not cause spinal cord injury but may cause segmental spinal nerve and/or cauda equina injuries. Injuries proximal to L1, above the termination of the spinal cord, often precipitate a combination of spinal cord lesion and segmental root or spinal nerve injury.

The spinal cord itself is organized into a series of tracts or neuropathways that carry motor (descending) and sensory (ascending) information. These tracts are specifically organized anatomically within the spinal cord.

The corticospinal tracts are descending motor pathways located anteriorly within the spinal cord.

The dorsal columns, located posteriorly, are ascending sensory tracts that transmit light touch, proprioception and vibration to the sensory cortex. They do not decussate until the medulla.

Pain and temperature are transmitted in the lateral spinothalamic tracts and usually decussate within three segments as they ascend.

Injury to the corticospinal tract or the dorsal columns results in ipsilateral paralysis and loss of sensation to light touch, proprioception and vibration respectively. As opposed to the other tracts, injury to the lateral spinothalamic tract will cause contralateral loss of pain and temperature sensation. Light touch is also transmitted within the anterior spinothalamic tract. Hence, injury to the dorsal columns may result in complete loss of vibration and proprioception but only partial loss of sensation. Similarly, anterior cord injury precipitates paralysis and incomplete loss of light touch.

Autonomic function traverses within the anterior interomedial tract. Sympathetic nervous system fibres exit from the spinal cord between C7 and L1, while parasympathetic system pathways exit between S2 and S4. Progressively higher spinal cord lesions cause increasing degrees of autonomic dysfunction.

Neurogenic shock is characterized by severe autonomic dysfunction, resulting in hypotension, relative bradycardia, peripheral vasodilatation and hypothermia. It does not usually occur with spinal cord injury below T6. Shock associated with these lower thoracic spinal cord injuries is haemorrhagic until proven otherwise.

The blood supply of the spinal cord is comprised of one anterior and two posterior spinal arteries. The anterior spinal artery supplies the anterior two-thirds of the cord. Ischaemic injury of this vessel results in dysfunction of the corticospinal, lateral spinothalamic and the autonomic interomedial pathways.

Urological complications of spinal cord injury

After spinal cord lesion a voiding dysfunction is present in most patients. This will express itself in various symptoms: disturbed or failing bladder sensation, failing or incomplete emptying, incontinence.

The acute phase of the spinal cord lesion is called 'spinal shock'. The bladder is able to store urine, but unable to void. Unless appropriate measures are taken, overflow incontinence with over-extension of the bladder and urinary tract infections will occur.

Following severe injury to the spinal cord the bladder becomes acontractile. With suprasegmental spinal injuries, the bladder gradually recovers its contractile function within months. Injuries to the sacral cord if complete enough may leave the bladder permanently acontractile. More often however these lesions are partial and a mixed degree of detrusor sphincter spasticity is found with a variable degree of weakness. During the spinal shock stage, some type of bladder drainage will require immediate attention. Chronic over-distension can damage the detrusor muscle and limit functional recovery of the bladder. Intermittent catheterization has proved to be the best form of management.

The aims therefore in the early phase of spinal cord lesion are prevention of early complications such as bladder over-distension, urinary tract infection, stone formation and urethral injury.

Bladder rehabilitation in spinal cord injury patients

Rehabilitation depends on classification of voiding dysfunction and assessment of risk factors. This can be determined by the clinical neuro-urological status of the patient and the use of video-urodynamics. (The timing of the urodynamic diagnosis depends on cause, location, and type [complete/incomplete] of the lesion, and on neurologic and neuro-urologic symptoms.)

Complete lesions

Areflexic bladder condition (lower motor neurone lesion)

It is important that bladder storage function under physiological compliance and capacity is maintained. If these cannot be achieved adequate incontinence care with low pressure and complete bladder emptying are optimal goals.

1. Diagnosis. No sacral sparing (complete loss of sensation in the saddle area, no voluntary anal sphincter contraction). No anal reflex or bulbo cavernous reflex (BCR).

Video-urodynamic characteristics will be:

- No sensation.
- Compliance seldomly decreased, no detrusor contraction, not even with physical or medical provocation.

- No sphincter contraction.
- Pelvic floor EMG without spontaneous activity.
- Bladder neck open or closed.

Hyperreflexic condition (upper motor neurone lesion)

The important features here are no sensation, detrusor hyperreflexia, and sphincter hyperreflexia.

1. Diagnosis

- Check voiding diary.
- Clinical neuro-urological status.
- No sacral sparing.
- Positive anal reflex and BCR.

2. Video-urodynamic findings

- Loss of bladder sensation.
- Uninhibited detrusor contractions.
- Detrusor sphincter dyssynergia (DSD).
- Low reflex volume.
- Normal or decreased detrusor compliance.

3. Risk factors

- Low compliance $<20\,\mathrm{ml/cmH_2O}$.
- High leak point pressure (LPP) (high pressure during storage phase).
- Low reflex volume with high residual urine.
- Maximal detrusor pressure in men $>80\,\mathrm{cmH_2O}$, in women $>60\,\mathrm{cmH_2O}$ (high pressure during voiding phase).
- Significant detrusor sphincter dyssynergia (DSD).
- Autonomous dysreflexia.
- Vesico-ureteral reflux.
- Influx into the male adnexae.

Autonomic dysreflexia (AD)

This is a condition that can occur in anyone who has a spinal cord injury at or above the T6 level. It is related to disconnections between the body below the injury and the control mechanisms for blood pressure and heart function. It causes the blood pressure to rise to potentially dangerous levels.

AD can be caused by a number of things. The most common causes are a full bladder, bladder infection, severe constipation or pressure sores. Anything that would normally cause pain or discomfort below the level of the spinal cord injury can trigger dysreflexia. Symptoms such as a pounding headache, spots before the eyes or blurred vision are the direct result of the high blood pressure that occurs when blood vessels below the injury constrict. The body responds by dilating blood vessels above the injury, causing flushing of the skin, sweating and occasionally goosebumps. Some patients describe nasal stuffiness and will feel very anxious. Uncontrolled AD can cause a stroke if not treated.

The treatment for AD involves removing the reason for the stimulation. One of the first things a patient can do is to sit up. This naturally decreases blood pressure.

If there is a catheter in place, it should be checked to be certain that there is not a kink in the tubing. If there is not a catheter in place, the patient should be catheterized. The bowels should be checked ensuring there is no stool in the rectum.

Measures for women and men with adequate hand function

- Intermittent self-catheterization (SIC) with anticholinergic therapy, anticholinergics are not necessary with high reflex volume or weak detrusor contraction ($<20\,cmH_2O$) in continent patients.
- Triggered reflex voiding, in men usually with sphincterotomy for DSD.
- Sacral deafferentation (SDAF) with implantation of a sacral anterior root stimulator (SARS), particularly after failed or instead of unwanted conservative treatment.
- For untreatable autonomous dysreflexia with hypertensive crises, spontaneous reflex voiding may be contra-indicated because of incontinence.
- Auto-augmentation is indicated if SDAF-SARS is impossible or unwanted, or when pharmacotherapy with intermittent catheterization (IC) has failed.
- Augmentation (enterocystoplasty) with IC is for organic low bladder compliance.
- Suprapubic catheterization (SC) or indwelling catheter (ID) with anticholinergic therapy is indicated only when other treatments are impossible.

Measures for women with inadequate hand function

- IC with anticholinergic therapy requires qualified nursing staff with high effort.
- Triggered reflex voiding exceptional at high reflex volume. Spontaneous voiding is not recommended.
- Sacral deafferentation (SDAF) with implantation of a sacral anterior root stimulator (SARS), particularly after unsuccessful, impossible, too nursing intensive, or unwanted conservative treatment.
- For untreatable autonomic dysreflexia with hypertensive crises, auto-augmentation when SDAF-SARS is impossible or unwanted, or with failed IC.
- Augmentation (enterocystoplasty) for organic low compliance bladder.
- This requires qualified nursing with high effort because IC is still needed.
- SC or ID with anticholinergic therapy is recommended when other treatments are impossible.

Measures for men with inadequate hand function

- Spontaneous reflex voiding with condom catheter drainage system (CCDS).
- Sphincterotomy is often necessary because of DSD.
- Triggered voiding in condom urinal.
- Sphincterotomy often necessary because of DSD.
- IC with anticholinergic therapy when CCDS is impossible or unwanted.
- Prerequisites: qualified nursing, high nursing effort (IC third party).
- SDAF + SARS when triggered voiding with sphincterotomy and other conservative treatments are unsuccessful or impossible.
- For untreatable autonomous dysreflexia with hypertensive crises, third party needed for emptying.

- Auto-augmentation only if SDAF-SARS is impossible or unwanted, or anticholinergic therapy with IC failed.

Incomplete lesion

Detrusor or sphincter or bladder neck may be normal, hyperreflexic or areflexic. Sensation may be normal or abolished.

Spontaneous recovery may be possible but it is important to start reversible treatment first and start a definitive treatment not earlier than 2 years after injury.

According to clinical conditions, incomplete lesions can be classified into three types:

1. Viscerosensoric (sensory).
2. Visceromotoric (motor).
3. Somatomotoric (sensory-motor).

Mostly combinations of the different types are present.

1. Viscerosensoric (sensory) incomplete condition

- Characteristics. Sensation of bladder filling is reduced and/or urge sensation delayed, 'too late', or excessive bladder sensation (caused by erroneous CNS control).
- Measures.
  (i) For reduced, delayed or too late bladder filling (urge) sensation, sensation is possibly ameliorated by neuromodulation (intravesical electrostimulation). Additional cholinergics are seldom needed.
  (ii) For excessive bladder sensation:
    - Neuromodulation (electrostimulation of pudendal nerve or sacral nerves).
- Medical treatment (anticholinergics, tranquillizer, local anaesthetics, prostaglandin synthesis inhibitors).
- Behavioural therapy.
- Bladder instillation with local anaesthetic or possibly capsaicin.

2. Visceromotoric (motor) incomplete UMNL

- Characteristics
  (i) Clinical
    - Voluntary initiation and/or inhibition of detrusor contraction.
  (ii) Urodynamical
    - Detrusor hyperreflexia with preserved urge sensation.
    - Disorder of voluntary initiation and/or inhibition of detrusor contraction possible.
- Measures on failure of inhibition of detrusor contraction
  (i) Conservative
    - Detrusor relaxant drugs (anticholinergics, combined with bladder drill).
    - Neuromodulation: (pudendal stimulation, sacral nerve stimulation).
  (ii) Surgical
    - Augmentation, if conservative measures fail.

- Measures on failure of initiation of detrusor contraction
  - (i) Conservative
    - Triggered reflex voiding which is seldomly combined with cholinergic drugs.
    - IC when combined with anticholinergic drugs.
  - (ii) Neuromodulation
    - Intravesical electrostimulation, sacral nerve stimulation.

3. *Visceromotoric (motor) incomplete LMNL*

- Characteristics
  - (i) Clinical
    - Incomplete voiding (residual urine).
  - (ii) Urodynamical
    - Detrusor hypocontractility.
- Measures
  - (i) Conservative
    - Cholinergics (bladder stimulants) combined with α-blockers (sphincter relaxants); or IC.
  - (ii) Neuromodulation
    - Intravesical electrostimulation, sacral nerve stimulation.
  - (iii) Surgical
    - Reduce outlet resistance (special video-urodynamic assessment is necessary before considering any operations).

4. *Somatomotoric (sensory-motor) incomplete UMNL*

- Characteristics
  - (i) Clinical
    - Delayed or incomplete or intermittent voiding.
  - (ii) Urodynamical
    - Incomplete or intermittent or failure of external sphincter or pelvic floor relaxation. The latter is confirmed by pelvic floor EMG. Reduced flow or intermittent flow despite detrusor contraction.
- Measures
  - (i) Conservative
    - Intermittent catheterization.
  - (ii) Medical
    - Antispastics (relaxation of striated muscles) not or little effect in tolerable dosage.
  - (iii) Surgical
    - Pharmacologic sphincter paralysis (local application of botulinum toxin); sphincterotomy (continence depending on competent bladder neck).

5. *Somatomotoric (sensory-motor) incomplete LMNL*

- Characteristics
  - (i) Clinical
    - Reduced anal sphincter tone and/or reduced voluntary contraction of anal sphincter.
    - Neurogenic stress incontinence.

    (ii) Urodynamical
- Hypotonic urethra and/or reduced contractility of striated sphincter/ pelvic floor muscles.
- Measures
    - (i) Conservative
        - Pelvic floor training.
        - Medical reinforcement of striated sphincter is not possible nowadays, α-adrenergics may induce improvement by increase of bladder outlet resistance.
        - If continence cannot be achieved, incontinence care should be emphasized.
    - (ii) Neuromodulation
        - Pelvic floor electrostimulation (vaginal, anal).
    - (iii) Surgical
        - Sling suspension, artificial sphincter, combined with intermittent catheterization.

Long-term care

Neurogenic voiding dysfunction is not a static condition but it follows its own natural history that can manifest in changes of the lower and upper urinary tracts (firstly functional, later morphological) and also may affect (mostly deteriorate) male sexual function. The aims of long-term care are to preserve or restore quality of life and life expectancy by controlling risk factors and patient-orientated life-long regular care.

All activities of daily life should be impaired as little as possible by the consequences of the bladder dysfunction.

A schedule of investigations is important in all SCI patients. A urinalysis should be performed every 2 months and ultrasonography and residual urines every 6 months.

There are a number of general risk factors.

- Febrile urinary tract infection.
- Recurrent urinary tract infection (more than two episodes a year).
- Hypertensive crises (related to autonomous dysreflexia).
- Increased residual urine ($\geq 100\,ml$ or $\geq 20\%$ of bladder capacity) on multiple measurements.
- Increase or new occurrence of urinary incontinence.
- Appearance or increase of voiding problems.
- Hydronephrosis (ultrasound).
- Change of bladder morphology (bulging, pseudo-diverticulae, concrements).
- Persistent abnormal laboratory findings (ESR, blood count, leucocytes, CRP, kidney function).
- Any indication of deterioration of kidney function.

Assessment of risk factors only by video-urodynamics

Some risk factors can be assessed only by video-urodynamics. It can reveal silent pathological changes which are not clinically observed over a long period. A high-pressure condition reveals:

- Low compliance in the storage phase.
- Hypercontractility in the voiding phase.
- Incomplete inhibition of hyperreflexia by anticholinergics.
- Significant detrusor sphincter dyssynergia.
- Ballooning of the posterior urethra.
- Vesico-ureteral reflux (VUR).
- Influx into the male adnexae.

Life expectancy and quality of life

Life expectancy and quality of life are decisively dependent on early starting and life-long consequently continuing of neuro-urological care. This requires the acceptance and cooperation of the patient and the medical team. If these prerequisites are met and depending on location and size of lesion, life expectancy is hardly impaired (e.g. motoric complete tetraplegics) or not impaired at all.

The decisive factor for life expectancy is the preservation of kidney function, for quality of life is a bladder function according to the patient's situation and demands of continence or control of incontinence.

STRESS INCONTINENCE

Prevalence

From the age of 35 approximately 16% of women suffer from urinary incontinence.

Commonly, symptom patterns are mixed with frequency and urgency of micturition. When incontinence occurs with activities, it is often referred to as stress incontinence.

Definition of genuine stress incontinence (GSI)

The involuntary loss of urine associated with a rise in intra abdominal pressure in the absence of a significant change in detrusor pressure.

Physiological basis

Incontinence in women, in such situations, is thought to be due to an intrinsic loss of urethral strength, which is often associated with urethral hypermobility.

Predisposing factors

- Childbirth.
- Obesity.
- Previous pelvic surgery.

History and examination

It is important to enquire whether there are any symptoms to suggest a mixed pattern of incontinence with detrusor instability, such as frequency, urgency, nocturia and urge incontinence. It is also important to exclude symptoms of bladder outflow obstruction (poor stream, incomplete emptying, hesitancy) and of urinary tract infection. An obstetric history and record of any previous pelvic surgery should also be taken.

Examination should include an assessment of the suprapubic region to exclude a palpable bladder, and pelvic examination to look for the presence of a cystocele or rectocele, to assess urethral hypermobility and to demonstrate stress incontinence on coughing.

Investigation

- MSSU to exclude infection.
- Pad testing where the volume of leakage is assessed by weighing a pad after exercise.
- Urodynamic studies. These studies will help to exclude detrusor instability and can also be useful in assessing urethral hypermobility and bladder neck descent when performed as video urodynamic studies (the combination of urodynamics with a contrast medium with simultaneous radiological screening of the bladder and urethra).

Classification

When assessed by video-urodynamics stress incontinence can be classified into three types.

Type I   Incontinence in association with a rise in intra abdominal pressure in the presence of a normally positioned urethra and bladder neck.

Type II   Incompetent bladder neck and urethral hypermobility.

Type III   Intrinsic sphincter deficiency. External sphincter weakness in the presence of normal bladder neck.

Management

1. Conservative

- Weight loss.
- Pelvic floor exercises.
- A number of exercises will help strengthen the pelvic floor musculature. These are best performed under the supervision of a dedicated physiotherapist and include:
  (i) Exercises.
  (ii) Vaginal cones.
  (iii) Electrical stimulation of pelvic floor.

It is important to remind women that these exercises will need to continue indefinitely to receive lasting benefit. However, at least 30% of patients can be expected to respond to simple measures as above.

2. Surgical.

Surgical treatment should be reserved for those who have failed a trial of medical therapy. The identification of detrusor instability does not prevent the use of the various surgical options. There are a number of different surgical procedures:

- Injection of bulking agents such as collagen or macromolecules.
  (i) Advantages. Minimally invasive cystoscopic procedure.
  (ii) Disadvantages. Long-term results not proven.
- Sling procedures. These can be either autologous slings of rectus sheath, fascia lata or vaginal wall, or can be new artificial suspensions with prolene mesh slings (TVT tm ethicon and SPARC tm AMS).
  (i) Advantages. Relatively minimally invasive. Can be performed under local anaesthetic (prolene types). Procedure of choice in Type III GSI.
  (ii) Disadvantages. Not the same extent of long-term data as for colposuspension.
  (iii) Results. New prolene sling procedures give excellent results, 85% cure rate, with minimal complications.
- Open colposuspension. There are two common open colposuspension procedures which differ only in minor points: Burch Colposuspension and Marshall Marchetti Krantz Procedure.
  (i) Advantages. Good long-term cure rates; 70–80% cure rates at 10 years.
  (ii) Disadvantages. Open surgery with increased post-operative pain and delayed recovery compared with more minimally invasive procedures.

Further reading

Artibani W. Pelvic Floor Reconstruction. *Eur Urol*, 2002; **42/1**: (Curriculum Volume pp 1–11).

TESTICULAR CARCINOMA

Introduction

Testicular germ cell tumours are relatively rare. Approximately two to three new cases per 100 000 males are diagnosed each year and most occur during the second and third decade. It also takes on a greater significance than numbers alone might suggest as it is one of the few solid cancers which is curable in the majority of cases, even when it has metastasized, with a crude overall 5-year survival rate in the UK of 90%.

Presentation and initial management

Most family doctors will rarely see a patient with a testicular malignancy. The majority of these patients present with an enlarged testicle or a lump in the testicle. Pain and symptoms of inflammation may also be features at presentation.

Patients presenting with a swelling in the scrotum should be examined carefully and an attempt made to distinguish between lumps arising from the body of the testis and other intrascrotal swellings. Those patients suspected of harbouring a testicular malignancy, that is, a lump in the testis, doubtful epididymo-orchitis, or orchitis not resolving within 2 to 3 weeks, should be referred urgently for urological assessment.

All patients will undergo an ultrasound examination of both testes, abdomen and chest X-ray. Blood should be taken for assay of the tumour markers α-fetoprotein (AFP), human chorionic gonadotrophin (hCG) and lactate dehydrogenase (LDH) before operation. One or more markers are raised in 75% of cases of teratoma and measurement is necessary for staging and follow-up. A CT scan of chest/abdomen and pelvis is mandatory as part of disease staging.

Primary surgical management

An inguinal orchidectomy with division of the cord at the internal inguinal ring is the primary surgical treatment. A testicular prosthesis may be inserted at the time of operation. If there is any doubt to the pathological diagnosis a frozen section may be obtained at the time. Sperm storage should be offered to men prior to orchidectomy who may require chemotherapy or radiotherapy at a later date.

Management of the contralateral testis

In patients with a remaining small testis (< 16 ml), and those with a history of maldescent, biopsy should be considered. Patients with biopsy-proven carcinoma in situ of the contralateral testis should be offered irradiation of the testis. All germ cell tumours, with the exceptions of spermatocytic seminoma, arise from carcinoma in situ (intratubular germ cell neoplasia) which is often demonstrable in the seminiferous tubules of the testis surrounding the tumour. Approximately 5% of men with testicular cancer have carcinoma in situ (CIS) of the opposite testicle. Carcinoma in situ is thought to progress to invasive GCT in 50–100% of cases and therapy should be considered.

Pathology of testicular germ cell tumours

1. Classification. Testicular germ cell tumours (GCTs) can be subdivided into seminomas and teratomas (non-seminomatous germ cell tumour: NSGCT), both of which must always be considered as malignant neoplasms. Seminomas consist of sheets and cords of relatively uniform cells which resemble primitive germ cells whereas teratomas exhibit a wide variety of appearances reflecting the potential of the tumour stem cell to differentiate along embryonic and extra-embryonic lines analogous to the fertilized ovum. The main classifications in common use are those of the British Testicular Tumour Panel and Registry (TTP&R) and the World Health Organization (WHO). Teratomas and seminomas have different clinical outcomes and require different clinical management, although in some instances it may be difficult to distinguish between poorly differentiated seminomas and teratomas. All teratomas including teratoma differentiated (mature teratoma), with the exception of epidermoid cyst, are capable of metastasizing and must be considered malignant.

2. Comparison of British (TTP&R) and WHO classifications

British	WHO
Seminoma	Seminoma
Spermatocytic seminoma	Spermatocytic seminoma
Teratoma	Non-seminomatous germ cell tumour
Teratoma differentiated (TD)	Mature teratoma
Malignant teratoma intermediate (MTI)	Embryonal carcinoma with teratoma (teratocarcinoma)
Malignant teratoma undifferentiated (MTU)	Embryonal carcinoma
Yolk sac tumour	Yolk sac tumour
Malignant teratoma trophoblastic	Choriocarcinoma

The pathological staging of the tumour (pT category) follows the 1997 UICC TNM classification.

- pT0   No evidence of primary tumour
- pT1   Tumour limited to testis and epididymis without blood or lymphatic vascular invasion
- pT2   Tumour limited to testis and epididymis with vascular invasion or tumour extending through tunica albuginea to involve tunica vaginalis
- pT3   Tumour invasion of spermatic cord
- pT4   Tumour invasion of scrotum

Staging systems and prognostic groupings have been employed to help the clinician plan treatment and follow-up. These are as follows:

I No evidence of disease outside the testis

IM As above but with persistently raised tumour markers

II Infradiaphragmatic nodal involvement

IIA Maximum diameter <2 cm

IIB Maximum diameter 2–5 cm

IIC Maximum diameter >5–10 cm

IID Maximum diameter >10 cm

III Supra and infradiaphragmatic node involvement

Abdominal nodes A, B, C, as above

Mediastinal nodes M+

Neck nodes N+

IV Extralymphatic metastases

Abdominal nodes A, B, C, as above

Mediastinal or neck nodes as for stage 3

Lungs:

L1 <3 metastases

L2 Multiple metastases <2 cm maximum diameter

L3 Multiple metastases >2 cm in diameter

Liver involvement H+

Other sites specified

Teratoma (NSGCT)	Seminoma
Good prognosis with all of:	
Testis/retroperitoneal primary	Any primary site
No non-pulmonary visceral metastases	No non-pulmonary visceral metastases
AFP < 1000 ng/ml	Normal AFP
hCG < 5000 iu/l	Any hCG
LDH < 1.5 upper limit of normal	Any LDH
56% of teratomas	*90% of seminomas*
5-year survival 92%	*5-year survival 86%*
Intermediate prognosis with all of:	
Testis/retroperitoneal primary	Any primary site
No non-pulmonary visceral metastases	Non-pulmonary visceral metastases
AFP > 1000 and < 10 000 ng/ml	Normal AFP
or hCG > 5000 and < 50 000 iu/l or	Any hCG
LDH > 1.5 and < 10 × upper limit of normal	Any LDH
28% of teratomas	*10% of seminomas*
5-year survival 80%	*5-year survival 73%*
Poor prognosis with any of:	
Mediastinal primary or non-pulmonary visceral metastases	*No patients classified as poor prognosis*
AFP >10 000 ng/ml or	
hCG >50 000 iu/l or	
LDH >10 normal	
16% of teratomas	
5-year survival 48%	

Disease management

Stage I seminoma of the testis without risk factors for pelvic node disease following inguinal orchidectomy is managed by prophylactic irradiation of the para-aortic nodes.

In patients with stage I teratoma or mixed seminoma/teratoma tumours of the testis surveillance is desirable in order to avoid possible treatment morbidity with adjuvant chemotherapy and is feasible because of the high chance of cure with chemotherapy on relapse.

Adjuvant chemotherapy should be offered to patients with stage I teratoma or mixed seminoma/teratoma of the testis following inguinal orchidectomy if high risk features are present (blood vessel and/or lymphatic invasion). This should be two courses of standard adjuvant platinum-based chemotherapy, that is, bleomycin, etoposide and cisplatin (BEP).

Management of metastatic disease

Metastatic seminoma is equally as chemosensitive as teratoma; this group of patients have increasingly been treated with chemotherapy, although there have been no randomized trials comparing chemotherapy and radiotherapy. Progression-free survival rates range from 85% to 100%.

Standard therapy for patients with metastatic teratoma should be four cycles of chemotherapy with bleomycin, etoposide and cisplatin.

Treatment of residual masses after chemotherapy

Surgery is usually only indicated for teratoma. Resection of seminoma is difficult and potentially dangerous due to lack of clear tissue planes and tumour infiltration beyond resection margins, and is limited to exceptional cases. Patients with teratoma who have residual masses after chemotherapy and whose markers have normalized should be treated by complete excision.

How often should patients be followed up?

Patients on surveillance are followed up monthly for the first year with clinical examination and serum markers at every visit. At present chest X-ray is performed at each visit and chest and abdomen CT at 3, 6, 9 and 12 months. In the second year follow-up should be 2-monthly with CT scans at 18 and 24 months. Subsequent follow-up should be 3-monthly for the third year, 6-monthly to the fifth year and annually thereafter to 10 years, with clinical examination, serum markers and chest X-ray at every visit.

Further reading

Rorth M *et al.* Carcinoma of the testes. *Scandinavian Journal of Urology and Nephrology*, 2000; **34**: 166–186.

TESTICULAR MALDESCENT

Testes should be within the scrotum at birth but spontaneous descent by 3 months to a year is more likely in babies with low birth weights or pre-term infants. After the first year of life, true testicular maldescent occurs in about 0.7% of boys. A recent study suggests that the number of boys with cryptorchidism (hidden testes) may be increasing and siblings of boys with undescended testes are at increased risk for cryptorchidism, with a reported incidence of up to 10%. Retractile testicles are rare before the age of 2 weeks but distinguishing retractile testicles from those truly undescended is important, as goals of treatment of undescended testicles include:

1. Enhancement of fertility.
2. Treatment of associated hernias.
3. Improvement of aesthetics.

The possibility of malignant degeneration in a patient with an undescended testicle does not reside solely with the testicle that is/was undescended. Malignant degeneration may occur in the contralateral so-called 'normal' testicle.

Imaging, such as ultrasound, CT scans and MRI scans, is generally not helpful.

It is important to differentiate between retractile testis, undescended testis and ectopic testis. Since a retractile testis does not require surgical intervention it is mandatory that this condition is diagnosed clinically. Retractile testis is due to hyperactive cremasteric reflex and the testis is pulled into superficial inguinal pouch or inguinal canal, when the child is undressed for examination. This is commonly observed at the age of 5 years or in a prepubertal boy. Retractile testis can be squeezed back into the fundus of the scrotum by an experienced clinician by a firm milking manoeuvre from the anterior superior iliac spine area towards the root of the scrotum. Incorrect diagnosis of retractile testis for undescended testis and ectopic testis in the past has led to undue claim by the clinician as having successfully treated undescended testis and ectopic testis by hormones.

Children with proven undescended testis and ectopic testis must be subjected to surgery before the age of 2 years. There is controversy with regard to an ideal age at which these children should be operated. With the current knowledge on the testicular histology and fertility index, it is sensible to advise surgery for a child born with an empty scrotum (unilateral or bilateral) if the testis is not found in the scrotum after his first birthday. The timing of orchidopexy is recommended for sometime before the age of 2 years because histologic changes in the undescended testicle begin at about 2 years of age with increasing fibrosis of interstitial tissue.

Anatomical considerations

A patent processus vaginalis and abnormal epididymis are commonly associated with undescended testicles. Moreover, when the processus vaginalis is patent, the ipsilateral epididymis is more likely to be abnormal. It is postulated that the patency of the processus vaginalis and epididymal maldevelopment are related to androgen deficiency.

Epididymal anomalies associated with cryptorchidism include agenesis, detachment of the caput or cauda epididymis, atresia, elongation with looping epididymis or vas, and widening of the mesentery between the testis and epididymis.

Anorchia may occur in 3–5% of boys operated on for cryptorchidism. Anorchia is unilateral in about 85% of these cases. The hCG stimulation test to document a testosterone surge has been shown not to be a reliable indicator of bilateral testicular agenesis. Extra and intraperitoneal exploration (when indicated) is still recommended for non-palpable testes.

Treatment options

At present, surgical treatment is advocated, in most cases, before the child's second birthday. This recommendation is based on two observations: spontaneous post-natal testicular descent is unlikely after this age, and histological abnormalities are subsequently more likely. Scrotal positioning also allows early detection of any testicular cancer, reduced risk of trauma and torsion, and improvement in germ cell function and ultimate prognosis of fertility.

The majority of parents opt for surgical treatment of undescended testicles because of the reasons outlined, such as the associated hernia, and also because they are unwilling to put their children through injections and the possible side effects of these hormones. Furthermore, because of the low benefit rate of hormonal treatment and the high success rate of single stage surgery, most children can undergo scrotal placement of testes by about 12 months of age.

Surgery is done under an outpatient general anaesthetic. The inguinal canal is opened and the testicle identified and dissected free. A passageway is made into the scrotum on the side of the affected testis, and a small scrotal incision is made. A small scrotal pouch is formed and the testicle placed within it and secured. The wounds are then closed with absorbable sutures.

Complications of surgery are unusual but may include testicular atrophy, retraction and hernia formation. Placement of an artificial testis in those in whom a testis is absent may be an option for some teenage boys, who may be self-conscious.

Outcomes

Semen quality may be impaired in men with a history of unilateral cryptorchidism, but reduction in paternity rates in these men has not been conclusively shown.

For men with a history of bilateral cryptorchidism, the prognosis for fertility is clearly worse and not proven to be improved by type or timing of treatment.

The risk of testicular cancer in men with a history of cryptorchidism has been adjusted downward in recent years. There now exists a relative risk of 4.7% in men with a history of cryptorchidism. This is essentially for intra-abdominal testicles, and this risk is not altered by orchidopexy. Approximately 15–20% of tumours occur in the contralateral descended testis.

Most tumours occurring in testes after previous successful orchidopexy are commonly non-seminomatous germ cell tumours, while those arising in abdominal testes are most frequently seminomas.

Recent studies have recommended non-intervention in patients older than 32 years with persistent cryptorchidism after weighing the risk of malignancy versus the risk of anaesthesia.

Further reading

Leissner D *et al.* The undescended testes: considerations and impact on fertility. *BJU International*, 1999; **83**:885–892.

TRANSITIONAL CELL CARCINOMA (TCC) OF THE UPPER URINARY TRACT

This condition is rare compared with TCC of the bladder (<5%) but has shared aetiological and clinical features. Recurrence is common (40%+) and virtually always distal to the original tumour. Contralateral synchronous or metachronous tumours occur in <3% of patients. Males outnumber females by 3:1 and the condition generally presents in the seventh decade of life.

Aetiology

- Cigarette smoking is the major factor.
- Occupational exposure to certain dyes and solvents.
- Analgesic abuse associated cancers and the entity of BALKAN uropathy are rare.

Presentation

- Loin pain.
- Haematuria (micro- and macroscopic).
- Sepsis.
- Metastatic features.

Investigation and diagnosis

1. Radiological

- Intravenous urography is the investigation of choice for patients with loin pain and frank haematuria. This will give anatomical and to some degree functional information.
- Ultrasound will reveal hydronephrosis but give no definite anatomical detail and may miss non obstructing tumours.
- CT scanning allows staging of ureteric and renal pelvic tumours.
- Virtual ureteroscopic reconstruction of helical CT is performed and this allows the user to navigate through the collecting system on a computer (at this time a ureteric catheter is required to inject contrast directly).

2. Urine analysis

- Cytological.
- Culture and sensitivity.

3. Endoscopic

- Cystoscopy to assess the bladder.
- Ureteric catheterization allows selective collection of ureteric aspirates for cytology and retrograde pyeloureterography further to delineate anatomical detail.
- Diagnostic ureteroscopy can be performed with either rigid or flexible instruments to allow direct visualization of any lesion and direct tissue sampling.

Differential diagnosis

- Blood clot.
- Radiolucent stone.
- Fungal ball.
- Sloughed renal papilla (analgesic abuse).
- Extrinsic compression (lymph nodes/blood vessels).
- Pyelitis/ureteritis (infection).
- Air (at retrograde pyelography).

Staging

The TNM staging scheme for upper tract TCC is given below. Recent work has shown that grade usually correlates with stage (96% G1 tumours have superficial disease) and this should be taken into consideration when defining treatment protocols.

Stage	Pathological findings
Ta, Tis	Mucosal disease
T1	Invades lamina propria
T2	Invades muscularis mucosae
T3	Extension through muscularis (into fat or renal tissue)
T4	Local spread to adjacent organs
N	Nodal disease
M	Metastatic disease

Treatment

- Open surgery
  (i) The gold standard (with normal contralateral kidney).
  (ii) Requires removal of the kidney and ureter along with a cuff of bladder (nephroureterectomy).
  (iii) Loin and either lower midline, extended gridiron or Pfannensteil incisions.
  (iv) The patient is then followed up cystoscopically as with bladder TCC.

If the tumour is in the renal pelvis or upper ureter the intramural ureter can be resected endoscopically and plucked from the bladder (this avoids two incisions). If the tumour is present in the distal ureter segmental resection has been described along with ureteric reimplantation.

- Mininally invasive therapy
- Laparoscopically assisted nephroureterectomy
  (i) Standard laparoscopic renal mobilization.
  (ii) The specimen is placed in the pelvis.
  (iii) The ureter is excised as with standard open surgery.

- Ureteroscopic electrocauterization
  (i) Well-differentiated, small volume disease.
  (ii) Abnormal renal function or a solitary kidney.
  (iii) Unfit for radical surgery.

Ureteroscopic electrocauterization or laser ablation of tumours <1.5 cm is acceptable but is associated with recurrence rates of 18–50%. Surveillence of the entire ureter is necessary as per bladder TCC.

- Percutaneous resection
  (i) Renal pelvic tumours.
  (ii) 50% recurrence rates.
- Adjuvant therapy in conservative surgery.

Mitomycin C or BCG can be instilled (either directly into the ureter via a single J stent or into the bladder with a double J stent in situ) and may improve recurrence rates. It should be noted that in all series the recurrence rate in the bladder is at 40%.

The follow-up of the contralateral kidney is not clearly defined. The presence of haematuria in the absence of bladder recurrences should alert the clinician to a further carcinoma.

Further reading

Clark PE, Streem SB. Endourologic management of upper tract transitional cell carcinoma. *Digital Urology Journal*. www.duj.com.

TUMOURS OF THE PENIS AND SCROTUM

Squamous carcinoma of the penis is a rare disease in the UK but is a significant health problem in some South American and African countries, where it may account for up to 20% of male cancers. Metastases from penile cancers spread by way of the penile lymphatics to the regional nodes, specifically the superficial and deep inguinal nodes, and subsequently the external iliac and obturator nodes within the pelvis. Involvement of the regional nodes with tumour is, in fact, the best predictor of long-term survival in patients with carcinoma of the penis.

Unlike cancers of the bladder, prostate and kidney, where metastases to regional lymph nodes portend incurable disease, penile tumours – like testicular cancers – may sometimes be cured by a regional lymphadenectomy. Approximately half of the patients presenting with penile cancers will have enlarged inguinal nodes. Since infection is often present, differentiation of inflammatory nodes from those involved with tumour metastases is frequently challenging. Between 30 and 50% of patients with palpable nodes will actually have metastatic cancer. More problematic are the 20% of patients with clinically negative groin nodes at diagnosis who have occult metastatic disease.

Without treatment, patients with metastatic tumour will die of their disease; no spontaneous remission of penile carcinoma has been reported. Therapy of such metastases, however, is prone to complications and frequently results in unpleasant side effects: penile and scrotal lymphoedema and substantial oedema of the lower limbs.

Given the high risk of such complications, one of the challenges of managing patients with penile cancers has been to determine which patients will benefit from inguinal dissection while avoiding unnecessary inguinal lymphadenectomies in patients without metastatic disease. The selection of those patients who should undergo ilioinguinal groin surgery has been an area of controversy for many years. However, an improved understanding of the natural history of penile carcinoma now permits a systematic and effective approach to management of these patients, based on the stage and grade of the primary penile lesion coupled with the status of the inguinal nodes at the time of diagnosis.

Clinical findings

Patients present with an indurated lesion, erythema or ulceration on the penis. As a result of this, patients may have bleeding, pain, discharge and obstructive voiding symptoms. The foreskin may obscure the lesion and up to a third of men may delay medical advice.

Laboratory findings are typically normal unless there is evidence of metastatic disease.

Penile carcinoma must be differentiated from other infectious lesions such as syphilis.

Pathology

1. Precancerous lesions

- Leukoplakia.
- Giant condylomata acuminata.

2. Carcinoma in situ. Bowen's disease. This is a squamous cell carcinoma in situ typically involving the shaft of the penis.

Erythroplasia of Queyrat. This is a velvety red lesion with ulceration which usually involves the glans penis. About a third of patients already have invasive carcinoma of the penis.

Staging and grading

Until recently, staging of penile cancers was by the Jackson system, first described in 1966.

- Stage 1. Tumours confined to the glans and prepuce.
- Stage 2. Tumours extending onto the shaft of the penis.
- Stage 3. Tumours with inguinal metastases that are amenable to surgery.
- Stage 4. Inoperable inguinal metastases or distant metastases.

A TNM staging system was introduced in 1972, and modified in 1987, and has become the standard system at present.

UICC Classification of penile cancer, 1987

	UICC , 4th edition, 1987
Primary tumour (T)	TX: primary tumour cannot be assessed.
	T0: No evidence of primary tumour.
	Tis: Carcinoma in situ.
	Ta: Non-invasive verrucous carcinoma.
	T1: Tumour invades subepithelial connective tissue.
	T2: Tumour invades corpus spongiosum or cavernosum.
	T3: Tumour invades urethra or prostate.
	T4: Tumour invades other adjacent structures.
Regional lymph nodes (N)	NX: Regional lymph nodes cannot be assessed.
	N0: No regional lymph node metastasis.
	N1: Metastasis in a single superficial inguinal lymph node.
	N2: Metastases in multiple or bilateral superficial inguinal lymph nodes.
	N3: Metastases in deep inguinal or pelvic lymph node(s), unilateral or bilateral.
Distant metastases (M)	MX: Distant metastases cannot be assessed.
	M0: No distant metastases.
	M1: Distant metastases.

Treatment of primary penile lesion

Biopsy of the lesion is important to establish a diagnosis. Lesions involving the prepuce can be treated with circumcision. Carcinoma in situ can be treated conservatively with Fluorouracil applications or Nd-Yag laser application. When confined to the glans, surgical excision of the affected glans and glans resurfacing has been recently adopted.

The goal of treatment of invasive lesions has been surgical excision. The use of primary radiotherapy, in the author's experience, is becoming less attractive because of potential complications of a scarred painful penis with associated urethral stenosis. Reconstructive procedures of the glans penis and penile shaft are available which allow adequate tumour excision and a functional penis. This has major plus implications for the psychological distress caused by partial or total penectomy. In those men not requiring reconstruction, a partial or total penectomy is advised. Enough functional length of penis is required for adequate voiding and sexual function in men undergoing a partial penectomy. A perineal urostomy combined with testicular excision and scrotal skin refashioning is advocated in men undergoing a total penectomy.

There is general consensus that patients presenting with superficial grade 1 lesions after treatment and palpably negative inguinal nodes may be followed expectantly. Similarly, there has been general agreement that patients with primary tumours of any stage and potentially resectable inguinal nodes which remain enlarged following a course of antibiotic therapy should undergo inguinal or ilioinguinal lymphadenectomy. Additionally, there is consensus that fixed inguinal nodes (stage T4) presage unresectable and incurable disease not amenable to surgical therapy. It is the patient who presents with invasive tumour but with clinically negative inguinal nodes who has presented the greatest therapeutic dilemma.

Considerations in inguinal and ilioinguinal lymphadenectomy

Because lymph node enlargement and lymphangitis due to infection of the primary tumour is common at the time of diagnosis, all patients with penile cancer should receive 4 to 6 weeks of antibiotic therapy before undergoing inguinal lymphadenectomy. At the completion of this course of treatment, the groins are carefully examined for the presence of abnormal nodes. Between 30 and 60% of patients who present with penile cancer have palpable inguinal nodes, and following antibiotic therapy, half of these nodes will harbour metastases. When metastases are detected clinically in one groin, contralateral metastases will be present in 60% of cases due to the crossover of lymphatics at the base of the penis. Consequently, in this situation contralateral inguinal lymphadenectomy should also be performed.

Prophylactic groin irradiation in patients having clinically negative groins has been investigated, and the incidence of subsequent inguinal metastases was found not to be reduced significantly by this treatment. Furthermore, irradiation makes subsequent physical examination of the groins difficult, and markedly increases problems with surgery and wound healing if a groin dissection later becomes necessary. Radiation may have a palliative role in the treatment of patients with unresectable disease, or in poor surgical candidates.

In the event of unilateral groin metastases developing some time after surgical treatment of the primary, inguinal lymphadenectomy of only the involved groin is required. While this would seem to contradict the recommendations outlined above, bilateral occult metastases which are present from diagnosis but which do not become clinically apparent until later should manifest themselves at about the same time. Consequently, the absence of clinically detectable nodes on the side contralateral to a late-developing groin metastasis suggests that the clinically negative nodes were not involved from the outset.

Preoperative staging of the pelvic, common iliac, and para-aortic nodes with CT scan and, where indicated, with needle biopsy, is essential. While survival has followed resection of tumour limited to the external iliac nodes, no patient with common iliac or para-aortic metastases has survived. Fine needle aspiration of suspicious nodes in these areas may confirm metastatic tumour and thus avoid unnecessary surgery. The most important predictor of ultimate survival continues to be primary tumour stage.

Occasionally, palliative groin dissection is performed even in the face of extensive regional or distant metastases. Lymphadenopathy which threatens to erode through the inguinal skin or invade into the femoral vessels may need to be removed to avoid pain, inguinal infection, or serious haemorrhage.

Sentinel node biopsy

The concept of the sentinel node postulates that there is a node or group of nodes – lying between the superficial external pudendal vein and the superficial epigastric vein – where the earliest metastasis from a penile tumour will occur consistently. A negative sentinel node biopsy in the presence of clinically negative groins was felt to indicate that further inguinal dissection was unnecessary. Five-year survivals of 90% have been reported in this setting. However, subsequent reports of the development of metastases following a negative sentinel node biopsy have suggested that sentinel node biopsy is not reliable. While further evaluation of this technique continues, most large centres treating penile cancer are no longer using it. Sentinel node biopsy is not appropriate in the presence of clinically suspicious nodes; rather full superficial and deep inguinal dissections should be performed. When the sentinel node biopsy is performed, the incision should be placed so that if a full formal inguinal lymphadenectomy is later required, the original sentinel node biopsy incision can be excised with the lymphadenectomy specimen.

Avoiding complications from inguinal lymphadenectomy

Despite the encouraging prognosis for many patients with inguinal metastases who undergo inguinal or ilioinguinal lymphadenectomy, there has been a long-standing reluctance on the part of surgeons to subject patients to this procedure because of the 30–50% incidence of major morbidity associated with it. Complications include: lymphocele, substantial lower limb lymphoedema, skin loss and infection. Skin flap necrosis can be minimized by selecting the appropriate incision, by careful tissue handling, by careful attention to skin flap thickness with excision of ischaemic flap margins, and by transposing the head of the sartorius muscle to cover the defect left over the femoral vessels. Lower limb lymphoedema can be reduced by careful attention to intraoperative ligation of lymphatics, by immobilization of the limb or limbs in the postoperative period, and by suction drainage of the lymphadenectomy site. Elastic support hose should be used in the immediate postoperative period and may be required long term in many patients. Wound infection can be minimized by intensive preoperative antibiotic therapy to reduce infection and inflammation from the primary, and by the use of prophylactic antibiotics. Thrombotic problems may be avoided through the use of subcutaneous heparin in the perioperative period, particularly when the classical inguinal and pelvic dissection is combined with prolonged bed rest post-operatively.

Conclusions

Surgery remains the primary treatment for squamous cell carcinoma of the penis, although combined approaches using chemotherapy and surgery are promising. Recent experience appears to confirm that an aggressive surgical approach utilizing immediate inguinal or ilioinguinal lymphadenectomy will improve survival in high-risk patients. Patients with low-grade, non-invasive disease and clinically negative groins who can be relied on to comply with follow-up may be followed expectantly. Patients having enlarged or suspicious nodes should undergo 6 weeks of antibiotic therapy followed by careful re-evaluation, and any residual suspicious inguinal nodes should be resected. High-risk patients, those with clinically negative groin nodes but grade II or III tumour or evidence of corporal invasion, should undergo immediate modified inguinal dissection, with full dissection if frozen section reveals metastatic tumour. Some patients with fixed inguinal nodal metastases may respond to neoadjuvant chemotherapy sufficiently to allow inguinal lymphadenectomy. Radiation therapy is not indicated for primary treatment nor helpful for adjuvant therapy, but may be useful as a palliative measure in late-stage unresectable disease.

Scrotal carcinoma

In the nineteenth century squamous epithelioma of the scrotum was the chimney sweep's cancer described by Percival Pott. With mechanization of the cotton industry, impure lubricating oil from the spinning machine soaking the crutch of the mule spinners' trousers proved even more carcinogenic than soot. Today a few cases of scrotal cancer occur in tar and shale oil workers but the majority of cases arise with no obvious aetiological factor. It is remarkable that, unlike carcinoma of the penis, carcinoma of the scrotum is almost unknown in India and Asiatic countries.

1. *Clinical features.* The growth starts as a wart or ulcer. As it grows it may involve the testis.

2. *Treatment.* The growth is excised with a margin of healthy skin. If associated enlargement of the inguinal nodes does not subside with antibiotics, a bilateral block dissection should be carried out up to the external nodes.

URETERIC CALCULI

Symptoms

- Loin pain.
- Scrotal or vulvar pain.
- Irritative lower tract symptoms.
- Haematuria.

Signs

- Loin tenderness.
- Occasionally testicular tenderness.
- Microscopic haematuria.

Investigations

1. Urine

- Analysis.
- Culture and sensitivity.

2. Blood

- Full blood count and differential.
- Urea and electrolytes.
- Calcium.
- Culture if patient febrile.

3. Radiology

- KUB plain radiogram.
- Shows up radiopaque calculi.
- Not good for small stones.

4. Ultrasound

- Renal stones.
- Distal ureteric stones viewed through bladder.
- Hydronephrosis.
- Ureteric jet may be seen in bladder on duplex scanning.

5. Intravenous urogram

- Anatomical and to some extent functional information.
- Current investigation of choice.
- Not good for small non obstructing stones.
- Caution
    - (i) Asthma.
    - (ii) Seafood allergy.
    - (iii) Diabetic (metformin). } contrast reactions
    - (iv) Poor renal function.
    - (v) The elderly.

- Non-contrast helical CT scan
  - (i) Will become the investigation of choice.
  - (ii) Currently higher radiation dose than IVU.
  - (iii) Higher diagnostic yield and sensitivity
    - Small stones
    - Lucent stones
    - Other pathology (GI system).
- Renography
  - (i) Functional information.
  - (ii) Useful in conservative management.

Management

- Signs.
- Symptoms.
- Size. ⎫ all contribute to management plan
- Sepsis.
- Economic factors. ⎭

1. Conservative

- 98% of stones <5 mm pass spontaneously.
- Spontaneous passage
  - (i) upper ureter 10%. ⎫
  - (ii) mid ureter 25%. ⎬ irrespective of size
  - (iii) lower ureter 50%. ⎭
- Minimal obstruction ideally.
- No sepsis.
- Symptoms controlled with simple analgesics.

2. ESWL

- Upper and distil ureter.
- Eswl in the pelvis is contraindicated in females of childbearing age.
- The ideal stone for lithotripsy is <1 cm.
- Not causing significant obstruction.
- In situ (no stent).
  - (i) Treatment of choice if available.
  - (ii) Stone clearance >85%.
- Ureteric drainage
  - (i) High grade obstruction.
  - (ii) Severe symptoms.
  - (iii) Sepsis.
- Percutaneous nephrostomy superior to ureteric stent for fragmentation and stone clearance
  - (i) Stent abolishes ureteral contraction.

3. Endoscopic

- Ureteric meatotomy.
- Blind electrohydraulic fragmentation. ⎫ historical
- Blind basket extraction. ⎭

4. Ureteroscopy

- First described in 1977 by Goodman.
- Initial instruments were of relatively large diameter(>13 Fr).
- Required dilatation of the ureteric orifice to pass into the ureter.
- Significant trauma in up to 25% of cases.
- Modern ureteroscopes are much smaller.
    - (i) Rigid.
    - (ii) Flexible.
- Rigid scope tapered to allow easy insertion
    - (i) Optics excellent.
    - (ii) Relatively large working channel.
    - (iii) Fibre optic bundles to transmit light and image.
    - (iv) Robust instrument.
- Flexible ureteroscope
    - (i) Very delicate and expensive.
    - (ii) In the best hands will last 20–30 uses.
    - (iii) Very useful in the difficult case.
    - (iv) Requires flexible instruments.
    - (v) Laser or electrohydraulic probes only.
- Procedure
    - (i) Cystoscopy and retrograde pyelogram.
    - (ii) Safety guide wire passed to kidney under fluoroscopy.
    - (iii) Ureteroscope inserted under vision.
    - (iv) May require second wire or ureteral dilatation (balloon). If access impossible stent inserted and return in 6 weeks.
    - (v) Flexible ureteroscope passed over a second guide wire under screening.
- Options when stone visualized
    - (i) Basket extraction under vision.
    - (ii) Stone fragmentation.
    - (iii) Electrohydraulic.
    - (iv) Ballistic
    - (v) Laser (gold standard). } with basket extraction
- Stenting postoperatively
    - (i) Trauma to the ureter.
    - (ii) Ureteric perforation.
    - (iii) Severe oedema of ureter.
    - (iv) Planned second look or eswl if stones have migrated.
- Antegrade ureteroscopy
    - (i) Indications
        - Impacted upper ureteric calculi
        - Failure to access from below.
    - (ii) Percutaneous puncture required (as per PCNL).
    - (iii) Flexible cystoscope used to visualize and fragment the stone.
- Rarely indicated.

5. Laparoscopic ureterolithotomy

- First described in 1994.
- Extraperitoneal or transperitoneal routes.

- Rarely indicated
  - (i) Large stones
  - (ii) Stones resistant to endoscopic fragmentation.
- The ureter is usually stented postoperatively and a drain left at the site of ureterotomy.

6. Open surgery

- Mainstay of management of ureteric calculi in the pre eswl/ureteroscopy era.
- Rarely performed nowadays.
- The ureter is approached via a grid iron incision.
- Extraperitoneal approach.
- Stone is removed via a ureterotomy after controlling the ureteric segment proximal and distal to the stone to prevent migration.
- The ureter is usually closed with absorbable suture material ± a ureteric stent and a drain left in the region of the ureterotomy.
- Compared with the previously mentioned techniques ureterolithotomy is associated with significant morbidity and requires longer convalescence.
- Indications
  - (i) Failed minimally invasive therapy where reconstructive procedure also necessary, e.g. ureteric reimplantation.

URETEROCELE

A ureterocele is a cystic dilatation of the distal end of the ureter within its intravesical segment. Most ureteroceles are part of a single renal system (orthotopic) but may also occur as part of a duplex system (ectopic ureterocele). In this case the ureterocele usually involves the ureter draining the upper moiety. The aetiology is still a little unclear but may be due to inadequate muscularization of the distal ureter or secondary to the dilatation of the distal ureter during development.

Presentation

Single system ureteroceles occur mostly in boys, but the ectopic ureteroceles are more commonly seen in girls. Most ureteroceles are now diagnosed at the time of fetal ultrasound. An ectopic ureterocele in girls may present as a prolapse through the urethra either as an intralabial mass or extending beneath the urethra and present between the labia. Before ultrasound the common mode of presentation was urinary tract infection and/or incontinence in the female with an ectopic ureterocele.

Investigation and management

Ultrasonography is the best initial step to diagnose a ureterocele. A voiding cystourethrogram and cystoscopy can confirm the suspicion of ureterocele. A renal scan is also required to assess the function of the upper tracts.

In single system ureteroceles the initial management is endoscopic incision. Vesico-ureteric reflux may occur, but if the kidney is salvageable a reimplantation may be performed. In ectopic ureteroceles the upper pole of the kidney tends to be dysplastic and without function. Treatment involves removal of the ureter and upper pole of kidney.

Outcome

Reflux can occur in up to 50% of ipsilateral ureters that are associated with ureteroceles. This may spontaneously resolve or require reimplantation.

URETHRAL STRICTURES

A urethral stricture is a scar and narrowing at one or more points in the urethra and of variable severity. This scar may compromise voiding and cause incontinence, bleeding, stones and even renal failure. This problem is almost invariably restricted to men and boys and is often secondary to injury (including catheter trauma) or inflammation. In many patients, no clear source of an event such as this can be recalled. Urethral strictures may be found in the urethra of women after severe pelvic trauma or after misguided urethral dilatations and over-stretching of the urethra.

The urethra's response to injury and/or inflammation and whether stricturing develops are extremely variable, as is the rapidity with which a urethral stricture develops after an insult.

Preventive measures

The most important preventive measures are in catheterization of the urethra, where even the slightest amount of trauma can lead to lifelong protracted problems with strictures. Therefore, it is imperative to be extremely gentle, liberally to instil into the urethra local anaesthetic jelly to both anaesthetize and lubricate the urethra, and to use the smallest possible silicone catheter necessary for the treatment. In addition, it should be removed as soon as possible. The catheter should also be changed in a timely fashion when left long term, and there should be no pressure on the penoscrotal junction.

Non-venereal and venereal inflammation may lead to strictures, so the judicious wear of condoms is appropriate in those facing this possible kind of exposure.

Evaluation

The most important test to evaluate and document the stricture is the retrograde urethrogram. This may be performed as an outpatient X-ray procedure for adult males, but in children it is ideally performed under an anaesthetic. This X-ray can then document the number and position of the various strictures as well as documenting the degree of stricturing. Furthermore, the stricture may be located in more than one position and can be found at the meatus or in the penile urethra, penoscrotal junction, proximal bulbous urethra, posterior bulbous urethra, membranous urethra or bladder neck.

Additional studies such as a voiding cystourethrogram, cystoscopy and biopsy in those in whom an irregularity is identified may be reasonable.

Treatment

Treatment options are extremely varied and provide some indication of the difficulty in guaranteeing a satisfactory result.

Watchful waiting

Watchful waiting can be undertaken if the patient is reasonably comfortable and can tolerate his symptoms without developing UTIs, voiding difficulty or leakage.

Procedures relying on regeneration of the urethral lining

1. Dilatation. This should be done gently with graduated sounds, careful generous lubrication and without over-stretching the urethra in addition to covering the patient with appropriate antibiotics. Self-dilatation is an option after the appropriate instruction. This is an option in which the patient may elect to do the urethral dilatations periodically himself as needed after the appropriate instruction.

2. Internal urethrotomy. This is usually done as an outpatient endoscopically, either blindly with the Otis urethrotome or through direct visualization with or without the aid of a camera, by incising the stricture and leaving a catheter in the bladder to allow healing about the catheter. The suggested length of time for leaving a Foley catheter draining after stricture treatment is extremely controversial and variable.

3. Buried strip. Buried strip such as that using the Denis Browne principle.

Anastomotic procedures

These are usually reserved for bulbous urethral strictures of 1 cm or less where the bulbous urethra can be reconstituted after excising the stricture and utilizing a 2-cm spatulated overlap anastomosis. Excised segments longer than 1 cm are likely to result in penile angulation.

Substitution procedures

1. Grafts

- Full-thickness skin grafts. Skin grafts using non-hair bearing skin may be harvested from several sites, including that from behind the ear.
- Bladder mucosal graft.
- Buccal mucosal graft. These urethral grafts used to repair strictures may be either unsupported or supported. The graft is spongiosupported when the spongiosum is used as a support to re-epithelialize the inner surface of the bulbospongy tissue.

2. Genital skin flaps

- Penile foreskin.
- Scrotal skin. The scrotal skin may be used as a flap if a sufficient area can be found without hair-bearing follicles; otherwise, this skin will need careful epilation.

Staged procedures

The first stage in a staged procedure focuses on opening the underside of the penis to expose the complete length of stricturing, securing these edges open to the external skin with or without various flaps and allowing the opened urethra, including its strictured area, to heal and mature over the succeeding months. During that time, the patient will void through this opened urethra.

The second stage is considered several months later, once the urethral area is soft and pliable and tubularization has a high likelihood of success. During this procedure, it will also be important to remove any hair follicles that may have been inadvertently included in the first stage of repair.

Urethral stents

These spiral-shaped devices are placed in the area of a stricture once it has been opened in an attempt to prevent restricturing. However, secondary inflammation has been a problem.

Further reading

Mundy *et al.* Urethral strictures and their surgical treatment. *BJU International*, 2000; **86**: 571–580.

URINARY FISTULAE

A fistula is an abnormal communication between two epithelialized surfaces. Vesicoenteric fistulae, also known as enterovesical or intestinovesical fistulae, occur between the bowel and the bladder. Vesicoenteric fistulae can be divided into four primary categories based on the bowel segment involved, as follows: (1) colovesical, (2) rectovesical, (3) ileovesical, and (4) appendicovesical fistulae. Normally, the urinary system is separated completely from the alimentary canal. Connections can occur as a result of (1) incomplete separation of the two systems during embryonic development (e.g. failure of the urorectal septum to divide the common cloaca), (2) infection, (3) inflammatory conditions, (4) cancer, (5) injury or (6) iatrogenically as a result of surgical misadventures.

The most common misconnection of the two systems occurs as a result of bowel disease that occurs adjacent to and erupts into the bladder. While fistulae also can occur from the bowel to the ureter and the renal pelvis, these occurrences are uncommon in the absence of trauma or surgical interventions. Fistulae may be either congenital or acquired (e.g. inflammatory, surgical, neoplastic). Congenital vesicoenteric fistulae are rare and often are associated with an imperforate anus.

Colovesical fistulae

A colovesical fistula is the most common form of vesicointestinal fistula and most commonly is located between the sigmoid colon and the dome of the bladder. The relative frequency of colovesical fistulae is difficult to ascertain because multiple disease processes and surgical procedures could be complicated by such fistulae.

The incidence of fistulae in patients with diverticular disease, the most common cause of colovesical fistula, generally is accepted to be 2%, although referral centres have reported higher percentages. Only 0.6% of carcinomas of the colon lead to fistula formation.

Colovesical fistulae occur more commonly in males, with a male to female ratio of 3:1. The lower incidence in females is thought to be due to interposition of the uterus and adnexa between the bladder and the colon.

Fistula formation is believed to evolve from a localized perforation that has an adhered adjacent viscus. The pathologic process is almost always intestinal. Pathologic processes characteristic to particular intestinal segments cause those segments to adhere to the bladder. Therefore, the location of the segment can suggest intestinal pathology.

Colovesical fistulae primarily result from diverticular disease. Ileovesical fistulae most likely are associated with Crohn's disease. Rectovesical fistulae occur more frequently in the setting of trauma or malignancy. Appendicovesical fistulae tend to be associated with a history of appendicitis.

Presentation

The presenting symptoms and signs of enterovesical fistulae occur primarily in the urinary tract. Symptoms include suprapubic pain, irritative voiding symptoms, and complaints associated with chronic urinary tract infection (UTI). Signs include abnormal urinalysis findings, malodorous urine, debris in the urine, haematuria and UTIs.

Pneumaturia and fecaluria may be intermittent and must be sought carefully in the history. Pneumaturia occurs in approximately 60% of patients but is non-specific because it can be caused by gas-producing organisms (e.g. clostridium, yeast) in the bladder, particularly in patients with diabetes (i.e. fermentation of diabetic urine), or in those undergoing urinary tract instrumentation. Pneumaturia is more likely to occur in patients with diverticulitis or Crohn's disease than in those with cancer. Fecaluria is pathognomonic of a fistula and occurs in approximately 40% of cases. The flow through the fistula predominantly occurs from the bowel to the bladder. Patients very rarely may pass urine from the rectum.

Investigations

Urinalysis usually shows a full field of WBCs, bacteria and debris.

Urine microbial culture findings are most commonly interpreted as mixed flora. The predominant offending organism is *Escherichia coli*. Attempts should be made to characterize the predominant organisms and obtain sensitivities to guide further therapy.

Anaemia may be present with chronic disease and may be associated with malignancy. Renal function tends to be normal.

Radiological investigations

A CT scan of the abdomen and pelvis is the most sensitive test for detecting a colovesical fistula and a CT should be included as part of the initial evaluation of patients with suspected colovesical fistulae. A CT scan can demonstrate small amounts of air or contrast material in the bladder, localized thickening of the bladder wall, or an extraluminal gas-containing mass adjacent to the bowel wall.

Barium enema imaging rarely reveals a fistula but is useful in delineating diverticular disease from cancer.

A cystogram may demonstrate contrast outside the bladder but is less likely to demonstrate a fistula.

Diagnostic procedures

Cystoscopy is an essential component of the diagnostic evaluation. This procedure can suggest the presence of a fistula and can allow evaluation for possible malignancy.

Exploratory laparotomy is diagnostic and therapeutic in all types of fistulae.

Histologic findings

Histologic findings associated with a biopsy of fistulous sites usually are consistent with chronic inflammation. Even in the case of carcinoma, inflammation is the usual finding on the bladder side. In more advanced cases, mucin-producing adenocarcinoma may be identified. The differential diagnosis must include primary adenocarcinoma of the bladder or poorly differentiated urothelial carcinoma. The clinical scenario and findings through laparotomy usually are helpful in determining the diagnosis.

Medical therapy

Non-surgical treatment of colovesical fistulae may be a viable option in select patients who can be maintained on antibacterial therapy for symptomatic relief for a prolonged period.

Enterovesical fistulae due to Crohn's disease may be managed conservatively with sulfasalazine, corticosteroids, antibiotics (e.g. metronidazole), and 6-mercaptopurine.

Patients with advanced carcinoma may be treated with catheter drainage of the bladder alone or supravesical percutaneous diversion.

Surgical treatment

Colovesical fistulae almost always can be treated with resection of the involved segment of colon and primary re-anastomosis. When the aetiology of the fistula is inflammation, the general principle is the resection of the primarily affected diseased segment of intestine with or without closure of the defect in the bladder. Healing of the bladder usually is uneventful and is allowed to occur with temporary urethral catheter drainage.

A diverting colostomy, with our without urinary diversion, may be used in cases of advanced cancer for palliation or severe radiation damage as a long-term solution.

Vesicovaginal fistula

Vesicovaginal fistula (VVF) is a subtype of female urogenital fistula (UGF). VVF is an abnormal fistulous tract extending between the bladder and the vagina that allows the continuous involuntary discharge of urine into the vaginal vault.

Aetiology

- Obstetrics – the usual cause is protracted or neglected labour.
- Gynaecological – the operations chiefly causing this complication are total hysterectomy and anterior colporrhaphy.
- Radiotherapy – the main cause is radiotherapy used in the treatment of carcinoma of the cervix; to a lesser extent external beam irradiation of the pelvic viscera for other reasons is responsible.
- Direct neoplastic infiltration – exceptionally, carcinoma of the cervix ulcerates through the anterior fornix to implicate the bladder.

When a wound of the bladder is recognized and repaired at once, leakage is uncommon, but escape of urine will quickly follow if such damage passes unnoticed. However, most vesicovaginal fistulas are the result of ischaemic necrosis of the bladder wall due to prolonged pressure of the fetal head in obstetric cases. In gynaecological cases, the ischaemia is brought about by grasping the bladder wall in a haemostat, including the bladder wall in a suture, or perhaps even by local oedema or haematoma. Leakage due to necrosis of tissue seldom manifests itself before 7 days after the operation.

An intractable fistula following radium treatment of carcinoma of the cervix uteri may arise from avascular necrosis years after the apparent cure of the original lesion.

Clinical features

There is leakage of urine from the vagina and as a consequence excoriation of the vulva occurs. Digital examination of the vagina may reveal a localized thickening on its anterior wall, or in the vault in the case of post-hysterectomy fistula. On inserting a vaginal speculum, urine will be seen escaping from an opening in the anterior vaginal wall. It is usually possible to pass a bent probe from the vagina into the bladder. Cystoscopy may be difficult, owing to the contraction of the bladder from cystitis and the escape of urine from the fistula. However, usually the tip of the probe that has been passed can be seen emerging through an area of granulation tissue.

Differential diagnosis between a ureterovaginal and vesicovaginal fistula can be made if a swab is placed in the vagina and a solution of methylene blue is injected through the urethra; the vaginal swab becomes coloured blue if a vesicovaginal fistula is present. With the advent of good, portable X-ray image intensifiers, a cystoscopy and bilateral retrograde ureterograms provide a more reliable demonstration of the anatomy. An IVU should be performed to exclude a coincidental ureterovaginal fistula. Usually it demonstrates some upper tract dilatation owing to partial obstruction.

Treatment

Occasionally, conservative management of a vesicovaginal fistula following hysterectomy by urethral bladder drainage is successful. Usually, operative treatment is required and the traditional teaching has been to delay surgery for some months. This has recently been questioned. The low fistula (subtrigonal) is best repaired per vaginam. The fistula is exposed with dissection of the edges which are freshened. The bladder is then closed using absorbable sutures and the vagina subsequently closed with a separate layer. A urethral catheter should be left in situ for at least 10 days. For the higher (supratrigonal) fistula, a transvaginal approach can be extremely difficult. These patients should always be cystoscoped prior to a repair procedure and bilateral ureterograms performed as occasionally one of the ureters is also involved. For the high fistula, a suprapubic approach is the best method in most hands. The Pfannenstiel incision should be re-opened, the bladder should be dissected free from the peritoneum and bisected posteriorly in the midline down to the level of the fistula. The bladder is then separated from the vagina and, occasionally, careful dissection from the rectum is also required. The vagina is then closed with a heavy absorbable suture and omentum brought down to lie between the closed vagina and the bladder anteriorly. This is lightly sutured in place and the bladder then closed. A urethral and suprapubic catheter should be left in situ for 10–14 days.

URINARY TRACT INFECTIONS (UTI) IN ADULTS

A UTI is an inflammation of the urinary tract by an infectious agent. Effective management begins by obtaining a careful history with attention given to current symptomatology, prior episodes of documented UTI, and risk factors that can initiate (e.g. urethral catheterization or sexual intercourse) or complicate (diabetes mellitus or pregnancy) a UTI. The higher incidence in females reflects the shorter urethra and lack of a prostate. The increased incidence in the teens represents urethral trauma due to sex; the general increase with advancing old age reflects obstruction, cystocele and atrophic vaginitis. Below age 50, UTI is almost entirely a disease of females.

History

The classical symptoms of UTI in the adult are dysuria with accompanying urinary urgency and frequency. A sensation of bladder fullness or lower abdominal discomfort is often present. Bloody urine is reported in as many as 10% of cases of UTI in otherwise healthy women; this condition is called haemorrhagic cystitis. Fevers, chills, and malaise may be noted; these usually are associated with upper UTI (pyelonephritis).

Pathogenesis

Pathogenesis of urinary tract infection involves complex interactions between an organism, the environment and the potential host. The majority of infections can be attributed to facultative anaerobes, the most common of which is *Escherichia coli*, which is responsible for 85% of infections in ambulatory patients and 50% of nosocomial infections. *Proteus mirabilis*, *Klebsiella* pneumonia and *Enterococcus faecalis* are the next most frequent isolates.

Most infections are caused by retrograde ascent of bacteria from the fecal flora via the urethra to the bladder and kidney. Haematogenous infection of the kidney by Gram-positive organisms, such as staphylococci, is possible though uncommon in normal individuals. There are urinary pathogen virulence factors that promote adherence to mucosal surfaces and subsequent infection. The bacteria usually express fimbriae or pili which mediate adherence to the epithelial cell receptors.

Host factors such as the epithelial cell receptivity are also important in the infection process. For example, *E. coli* bound to vaginal epithelial cells from healthy controls less avidly than to vaginal epithelial cells from women with recurrent UTIs. This binding specificity correlated with binding to buccal mucosal cells, suggesting a genetic predisposition to urinary tract infection. Vaginal cell receptivity also varies as a function of hormonal status. Bacterial adherence has been shown to be higher earlier in the menstrual cycle and in postmenopausal women as compared with premenopausal women or postmenopausal women who are on oestrogen replacement therapy.

On examination

1. Cystitis. Most adult women with simple lower UTI have suprapubic tenderness with no evidence of vaginitis, cervicitis, or pelvic tenderness (e.g. cervical motion tenderness, which suggests pelvic inflammatory disease). The patient may appear uncomfortable but not toxic.

2. Pyelonephritis. With pyelonephritis the patient usually appears ill and, in addition to fever, sweating, one may find costovertebral angle (flank) tenderness. The clinician may also appreciate signs of dehydration, such as dry mucous membranes and tachycardia, as well as poor vascular tone due to Gram-negative bacteraemia, which may be manifested by clammy extremities and profound orthostatic hypotension.

Initial investigations

Urine should be carefully collected in order to minimize contamination by non-pathogens and sent for microscopic analysis and culture. A midstream voided specimen is generally adequate, but urethral catheterization or suprapubic aspiration may be necessary in an individual who cannot produce a clean specimen. Since UTI is a host inflammatory response to bacterial invasion, urinalysis will reveal pyuria (the presence of white blood cells in the urine) and bacteriuria. If there is bacteriuria with no pyuria in an asymptomatic patient, an infection is not present and therapy is usually not necessary. Urine is normally sterile and traditionally 10^5 colony forming units per millilitre (cfu/ml) has been considered to be diagnostic of UTI. Frequent voids will reduce bacterial counts to less than 10^5 in 30% of patients with UTI. Therefore urine culture which shows growth of 1000 or more cfu/ml should be investigated in symptomatic patients. Culture and antibiotic susceptibility testing is not required for uncomplicated infection, but is essential to guide drug selection for complicated UTIs.

Treatments

Trimethoprim, a drug that interferes with folate metabolism, is frequently used in the treatment of uncomplicated urinary tract infections. With the notable exceptions of *Pseudomonas* and *Enterococcus* species, trimethoprim is effective against a broad range of urinary pathogens. Concentration of this economical drug in the urinary tract is excellent and the effect on the fecal flora is minimal. Use of this drug in pregnancy and neonates under one month of age is contraindicated.

Nitrofurantoin disrupts carbohydrate metabolism and inhibits bacterial cell wall synthesis. It is effective against most uropathogens except *Pseudomonas* and *Proteus*. Since nitrofurantoin reaches high levels in the urine, but does not concentrate in tissue, it is ineffective in the treatment of infection involving solid organs such as pyelonephritis or prostatitis. There is limited interaction with the fecal reservoir resulting in minimal problems with resistance. It should not be used in patients with poor renal function because they have insufficient concentrating ability to deliver adequate levels to the urinary tract or as initial therapy in patients with complicated UTIs.

Aminopenicillins (i.e. ampicillin and amoxicillin) are frequently used in the treatment of a wide range of infectious processes including those in the urinary tract. This frequent use has resulted in up to 30% resistance that can be seen in clinical isolates. Extended spectrum synthetic penicillins and those compounded with beta-lactamase inhibitors are occasionally used in parenteral therapy for complicated pyelonephritis.

Aminoglycosides, which inhibit bacterial RNA synthesis, are a useful class of drugs and, when combined with ampicillin, are part of first-line therapy against pyelonephritis. They have largely maintained their spectrum of activity and, with appropriate monitoring of levels, the danger of renal toxicity can be minimized.

Management

1. Lower tract infection. Cystitis, an infection of the urinary bladder, affects between 4–6 million women each year and it is estimated that over 25% of women in the 20–40 age group have had a urinary tract infection. Most infections in women are uncomplicated, whereas in men complicated infections predominate. The history should identify those with other processes causing similar symptoms such as vaginosis, urethral syndromes, sexually transmitted diseases, or other non-inflammatory processes. A presumptive diagnosis of acute bacterial cystitis can be made based on a thorough history and after urinalysis reveals pyuria and bacteriuria. Indirect dip-stick test for nitrite or leukocyte esterase is less sensitive. The threshold of 10^5 cfu/ml, usually considered to be diagnostic of UTI, should be lowered to 10^2 cfu/ml in patients who have symptoms consistent with UTI.

Choice of appropriate therapy is guided by whether the infection is complicated vs. uncomplicated, nosocomial vs. community acquired, as well as the sex of the patient. For uncomplicated acute bacterial cystitis in women, a 3-day course of trimethoprim is adequate empiric treatment. Fluoroquinolones should be reserved for patients with recurrent infections. The rational for antibiotic therapy in male patients is similar, although the duration of therapy should be 7 days.

Recurrent infections of the lower tract are likely to originate from outside the urinary tract. Obtaining an accurate history of prior infecting organisms, hormonal status, relationship of infection to sexual intercourse, and diaphragm or spermacide are all important. Radiologic evaluation of the upper tract is not indicated in otherwise healthy patients unless there is unexplained haematuria, obstructive symptoms, neurogenic bladder dysfunction, or diabetes. Cystoscopy is indicated in those with frequent infections and symptoms of obstruction, bladder dysfunction or fistula. Patients who have rapidly recurrent infections with the same organism should be evaluated to identify a focus of bacterial persistence, such as a calculus or ureteropelvic junction obstruction, which must be removed or corrected to prevent further episodes.

Prophylactic antibiotics are used to prevent re-infection from outside the urinary tract. This is in distinction to suppressive therapy which is used to repress a focus of bacterial persistence. Suppressive therapy is reserved for patients who cannot be rendered free of the focus of persistence or are poor candidates for such treatment. The basis for prophylaxis is the eradication of pathogenic bacteria from anatomic reservoirs (vaginal introitus and faeces) without promoting bacterial resistance. A single bedtime dose of nitrofurantoin (50 mg), 100 mg of trimethoprim, or cephalexin (250 mg) are all effective choices. Duration of therapy should be 6 to 12 months. If the patient experiences a symptomatic infection while on prophylaxis, full therapeutic dosing with the agent or another drug should be instituted, returning to the usual regimen after completion of the full course.

Other approaches to prophylaxis are also being investigated. In postmenopausal women, topical oestrogen replacement has been shown to restore the vaginal pH to its premenopausal range, promote recolonization with lactobacilli, decrease colonization with *E. coli*, and subsequently result in fewer infections.

2. Upper tract infection. Acute pyelonephritis or inflammation of the kidney parenchyma and renal pelvis is a clinical diagnosis made on the basis of the classic symptoms of fever, chills and flank pain. Other non-specific symptoms such as abdominal pain, nausea, vomiting or diarrhea can accompany acute pyelonephritis. Therefore, a high index of suspicion must be maintained to make prompt diagnosis. Urine culture shows *E. coli* in 80% of cases, with *Proteus, Enterobacter, Pseudomonas, Serratia* and *Enterococcus* also being common pathogens. Imaging studies, such as intravenous pyelogram, ultrasound, or CT scan are useful to rule out obstruction or focus of infection (e.g. abscess) that requires drainage. If the patient has a fever for longer than 3 days, is extremely ill, develops signs or symptoms of obstruction, or does not respond to initial antibiotic therapy, imaging studies should also be obtained.

Further reading

Stapleton A. Prevention of recurrent urinary tract infections in women. *Lancet*, 1999; Jan **2:353(9146)**: 7–8.

URINARY TRACT INFECTIONS (UTI) IN CHILDREN

The urinary tract is a relatively common site of infection in infants and young children. Urinary tract infections (UTIs) are more common in girls except during the first few months of life. Up to 1.5% of boys and 5% of girls develop UTIs during the school years. UTIs are important because they can cause acute morbidity and may result in long-term medical problems, including hypertension and reduced renal function. Management of children with UTI involves repeated patient visits, use of antibiotics and exposure to radiological investigations. Vesicoureteral reflux is the most commonly associated abnormality, and reflux nephropathy is an important cause of end-stage renal disease in children and adolescents. However, when reflux is recognized early and managed appropriately, renal insufficiency is rare. Some children who present with an apparently uncomplicated first urinary tract infection turn out to have significant reflux. Subclinical infections can sometimes lead to severe bilateral renal scarring. Therefore, even a single documented urinary tract infection in a child must be taken seriously. Accurate diagnosis is therefore extremely important for two reasons: to permit identification, treatment and evaluation of the children who are at risk for kidney damage and to avoid unnecessary treatment and evaluation of children who are not at risk, for whom interventions are potentially harmful and provide no benefit.

Diagnosis

Children with urinary tract infections do not always present with symptoms such as frequency, dysuria or flank pain. Infants may present with fever and irritability or other subtle symptoms, such as lethargy. Older children may also have non-specific symptoms, such as abdominal pain or unexplained fever. A urinalysis should be obtained in a child with unexplained fever or symptoms that suggest a urinary tract infection. In young children with urinary tract infections, urinalysis may be negative in 20% of cases.

Associated factors known to predispose to the development of UTIs

1. Age. There is an increased incidence of recurrent UTIs in the five year of life. This is secondary to the bacterial colonization of the periurethral areas in both girls and boys. It is unusual for these infections to continue beyond the age of 5 years.

2. Vesicoureteric reflux. Children with reflux have an increased incidence of UTI. Infants (up to 2 years) and young children are at higher risk than are older children for incurring acute renal injury with UTI. The incidence of vesicoureteral reflux (VUR) is higher in this age group than in older children, and the severity of VUR is greater, with the most severe form (with intrarenal reflux or pyelotubular backflow) virtually limited to infants.

3. Voiding difficulties. Some children have symptoms of bladder instability, such as urge incontinence or squatting behaviour, in the absence of an infection. Bladder instability may be improved by placing the child on a timed voiding schedule of once every 3h. Residual urines may predispose to UTIs. If behavioural approaches fail, voiding symptoms often respond to anticholinergic agents such as oxybutynin (Ditropan), in a dosage of 0.15mg per kg three times daily.

4. Constipation. This can lead to problems with bladder emptying and residual urines. Uncircumcised males: the rate of UTI in circumcised boys is low, 0.2% to 0.4%.The literature suggests that the rate in uncircumcised boys is 5–20 times higher than in circumcised boys. A resurgence of sentiment favouring routine neonatal circumcision has therefore occurred. Because of the data demonstrating an increase in the rate of infection, routine circumcision has been advocated by some authors. They point out the significant mortality and renal scarring associated with urinary tract infections occurring in early infancy. However, circumcision is a permanent solution to a problem that affects males only during the first 6 months of life. There may be alternative, non-surgical means of preventing these infections, and the question of whether all boys should be circumcised to prevent infection in 1–4% remains debatable. It is also unclear whether circumcision would augment the benefit of antibiotic prophylaxis in boys with reflux or other urological anomalies.

5. Anatomical abnormalities. Any urological abnormality which causes problems with drainage of the urinary tract may predispose to UTIs. Examples are pelviureteric obstruction, ureterovesical obstruction or posterior urethral valves in boys.

The most reliable method of obtaining urine for a culture is suprapubic aspiration. This procedure, however, often causes anxiety in the child, the parent and the doctor. Urine specimens may therefore be obtained by placing a plastic bag over the perineum of infants, and by obtaining a voided specimen in older children. Because 'bagged' and voided specimens may be contaminated, results must be interpreted in conjunction with the urinalysis and the clinical setting. Pyuria and/or classic symptoms support the diagnosis of a urinary tract infection, whereas a positive culture in a child with a normal urinalysis and/or atypical symptoms may represent contamination. In patients whose diagnosis is complicated, and when the uncertainty of contamination must be avoided, a catheterized or suprapubic specimen can be obtained.

Of the components of urinalysis, the three most useful in the evaluation of possible UTI are:

1. Leukocyte esterase test. A positive result on a leukocyte esterase test seems to be as sensitive as the identification of WBCs microscopically, but the sensitivity of either test is so low that the risk of missing UTI by either test alone is unacceptably high

2. Nitrite test. The nitrite test has a very high specificity and positive predictive value when urine specimens are processed promptly after collection. Using either a positive leukocyte esterase or nitrite test improves sensitivity at the expense of specificity; that is, there are many false-positive results.

3. Urine microscopy. The wide range of reported test characteristics for microscopy indicates the difficulty in ensuring quality performance; the best results are achieved with skilled technicians processing fresh urine specimens.

The urinalysis cannot substitute for a urine culture to document the presence of UTI, but the urinalysis can be valuable in selecting individuals for prompt initiation of treatment while waiting for the results of the urine culture. The number of bacteria that must be present to cause a significant urinary infection is 10 000 to 100 000 colony-forming units/ml of voided urine. Any of the following are suggestive (although not diagnostic) of UTI: positive result of a leukocyte esterase or nitrite test, more than five white blood cells per high-power field of a properly spun specimen, or bacteria present on an unspun Gram-stained specimen.

Radiological imaging

Imaging of the urinary tract is recommended in every febrile infant or young child with a first UTI to identify those with abnormalities that predispose to renal damage. Imaging should consist of urinary tract ultrasonography to detect dilatation secondary to obstruction and a study to detect VUR.

When a child is screened for reflux (VUR), the appropriate test to obtain is a cystogram. Although renal ultrasound examinations are less invasive, they are normal in 50–75% of patients with reflux and, therefore, ineffective for screening. A DMSA renal scan is the best study for detecting renal scarring and might therefore identify patients at particular risk for reflux. Unfortunately, a renal scan will not detect reflux in children who have not yet developed scarring, and these are the very ones who might benefit most from antibiotic prophylaxis.

Two types of cystogram are available. A standard voiding cystourethrogram (VCUG) is obtained by instilling radiopaque contrast medium into the bladder and imaging the bladder and renal fossae during filling and voiding. The severity of vesicoureteral reflux is graded depending on the degree of distension of the collecting system.

A nuclear cystogram can be obtained by instilling a radionuclide agent into the bladder and imaging with a gamma camera. Nuclear cystography is at least as sensitive for the detection of reflux as a standard VCUG and exposes the child to less radiation. However, grading of reflux is less precise, and associated bladder abnormalities cannot be detected with nuclear cystography.

Treatment

Because urinary tract infections are usually caused by Gram-negative rods, particularly *Escherichia coli*, any oral antibiotic with good Gram-negative coverage is a reasonable choice for treatment. Trimethoprim offers good coverage. It is given in suspension form in a dosage of 4 mg trimethoprim per kg twice daily. Other commonly used antibiotics include amoxicillin, in a dosage of 10 mg per kg three times daily, and nitrofurantoin in a dosage of 2.5 mg per kg three times daily. Cephalosporins may be indicated if infection with a more resistant organism is suspected.

Children who require hospitalization should be placed on broad-spectrum intravenous antibiotics pending the results of the urine culture. Because most community-acquired urinary tract infections are caused by Gram-negative bacilli, coverage should include an aminoglycoside, a cephalosporin or a broad-spectrum penicillin derivative.

Recurrent UTIs

Children with frequent infections are managed with antibiotic prophylaxis administered in the same fashion as in patients with vesicoureteral reflux.

However, in the absence of reflux, upper tract monitoring and routine urine cultures are rarely indicated. Treatment of asymptomatic bacteriuria in this setting is unnecessary.

Further reading

Riccabona *et al.* Management of recurrent UTI and VUR in Children. *Current Opinions in Urology*, 2000.

URODYNAMICS

Urodynamics is the study of urinary tract function and dysfunction with two main specific aims; to reproduce the patient's symptomatic complaints and to provide a pathophysiological explanation for the patient's problems. A full urodynamic investigation consists of: (1) free-flow rate assessment; (2) measurement of post-void residual urine; (3) filling cystometry; and (4) pressure-flow study. These should proceed in the order described and each part of the study should be considered an integral part of the investigation, information provided from each section being collated with all others to give an accurate, objective evaluation of lower tract function.

Free-flow rate assessment

Free-flow rate assessment can be considered an initial tool for evaluating male patients presenting with lower urinary tract symptoms (LUTS), particularly symptomatic BPH. Uroflowmetry can provide valuable information over symptoms alone in diagnosing the cause of lower tract dysfunction, providing performance statistics for maximum and average flow rate. This may obviate the need for formal urodynamic study in routine clinical practice. Useful information can also be obtained by observing the flow pattern itself – the characteristic bell-shaped curve in the normal male, converting to the prolonged, oscillating trace pathognomonic of bladder outflow obstruction (BOO) or the low amplitude plateau, suggesting urethral stricture. Free-flow rate assessment is limited, however, by an inability to discriminate between low flow due to BOO or impaired detrusor function.

Post-void residual urine

Post-void residual urine is usually performed either by catheterization or ultrasonic scanning. When investigating BOO, a residual urine volume exceeding 100 to 150 cc is considered significant. It must be borne in mind, however, that the presence of residual urine is not caused only by BOO per se and that patients with BOO may present insignificant residual urine because of compensatory mechanisms, such as detrusor hypertrophy or abdominal straining to facilitate bladder emptying.

Filling cystometry

The filling cystometry method objectively quantifies the storage function of the lower urinary tract. It is used to assess detrusor activity, sensation, capacity, compliance and urethral competence.

The normal bladder should be stable under all conditions of filling or stress. The compliance of the bladder (Change Vol/P) is also of interest as is its capacity and the patient's sensations of strength of desire to void. Two pressure channels are typically measured, rectal pressure and bladder (intravesical). The rectal pressure responds to any changes of the abdominal cavity due to straining or stress. These can then be subtracted from the intravesical to give the true intrinsic bladder pressure from the detrusor muscle (detrusor pressure).

Quality control is important during cystometry. The cancellation from the rectal catheter must be accurate. Earlier methods employing bladder insufflation with gas have been superseded by infusing isotonic fluids at fill rates ranging from 30 cc/min to 120 cc/min.

1. **Fast fill cystometry.** A rate of 100 ml/min is used and intended to provoke any underlying detrusor dysfunction such as detrusor instability.

2. **Medium flow cystometry.** A rate of 30–60 ml/min is used and recommended as an alternative to fast flow filling in patients known to have hypersensitive bladders associated with irritative symptoms and pain.

3. **Slow fill cystometry.** A rate of 10–20 ml/min is used and recommended in patients known to suffer with detrusor instability or hyperreflexia. This fill rate is intended to mimic physiological filling.

Urodynamic parameters provided by this method include subjectively perceived volumes at first sensation of bladder filling, first desire to void, strong desire to void, urgency and maximum cystometric capacity. Filling cystometry also measures detrusor pressures throughout the filling phase. The International Continence Society (ICS) although not providing numerical values has standardized the terminology for urodynamic diagnoses. During the filling phase these are as follows:

1. The stable detrusor is one that does not contract during the filling phase while the patient is attempting to inhibit micturition.
2. The unstable detrusor is one that is shown to contract spontaneously or on provocation during the filling phase while the patient is attempting to inhibit micturition.

Hyperreflexia is defined as overactivity due to disturbance of the nervous control mechanism. This term should only be used where there is objective evidence of neurological disorder.

During the filling phase the urethra maintains a positive closure pressure. Leakage of urine however in the absence of a detrusor contraction is termed 'genuine stress incontinence' (GSI).

Voiding studies

Voiding studies are used to assess detrusor contractility and urethral obstruction. The urodynamic parameters of relevance during the voiding phase include maximum urinary flow rate (Qmax); average urinary flow rate; time to reach Qmax and detrusor pressure at various corresponding flow rates, particularly the detrusor pressure at Qmax (PdetQmax). From such parameters, the degree of BOO can be classified using specific normograms. To obtain optimum results, the study should be performed with a small catheter, to prevent flow obstruction artifact.

Abnormally high voiding pressure indicates outflow tract obstruction when associated with a low initial flow rate. High flow rates, in excess of 40 cc/s, may be associated with exceptionally powerful detrusor contractions and higher than normal voiding pressure, in both sexes. This is most often seen in patients with long-standing bladder overactivity and detrusor hypertrophy, but no outflow obstruction. In women, voiding commonly occurs with a low voiding pressure. The detrusor may be proven to be contracting by measuring the isometric pressure on interruption of flow. A poorly sustained voiding pressure may be related to a failing detrusor. An unsustained contraction is likely to lead to residual urine.

Ambulatory urodynamics

This technique is used in more specialized units for complex cases. It is particularly helpful where monitoring needs to span longer time periods such as identifying the cause of nocturnal enuresis. The equipment is patient-controlled and the information downloaded to a computer source at the end of the procedure.

Video urodynamics

This requires the availability of the most specialized urodynamic equipment. The digital monitoring systems take video image information from a fluoroscopy unit and provide digital video image, on screen with pressure data. This process allows the physician to visualize events in the lower urinary tract along with pressure, flow and EMG data.

In conclusion, the principal investigations are:

Investigation	Symptoms	Possible diagnosis
Uroflow	Frequency, nocturia, poor flow	Bladder outlet obstruction
Pressure flow	Frequency, nocturia, poor flow	Bladder outlet obstruction
Cystometry	Frequency, urgency	Detrusor instability
Urethral closure pressure	Incontinence	Genuine stress incontinence
Ambulatory urodynamics	Frequency, urgency pointing to unstable bladder but not shown on static urodynamics	Detrusor instability, Genuine stress incontinence

Further reading

Abrams P. *Urodynamics*. London: Springer, 1997.

UROLOGICAL RECONSTRUCTION

Recent advances in surgical technique, the successful application of intermittent catheterization to the reconstructed urinary tract, and the lessons learned from the pioneering work on urinary undiversion have allowed patients to be reconstructed for continence as well as for preservation of renal function. Such reconstructive principles may now be applied to virtually all urinary tract anomalies with a good expectation for success. Reconstructive options are now available even for those patients with end-stage renal disease for whom renal transplantation will ultimately be required. The goals of reconstructive surgery are a large bladder capacity and a low pressure reservoir. These will help to ensure continence as well as a protective influence on the upper urinary tract. Adequate bladder outlet resistance must be provided to prevent incontinence, hopefully without sacrificing the potential for spontaneous voiding. Access for a quick, easy and painless catheterization is also critical.

Urinary diversion (incontinent)

This form of urological reconstruction allows for an incontinent conduit to be constructed. The ureters are anastomosed to the base of the conduit and the distal end forms a stoma. The commonly used intestinal segments used are terminal ileum and colon. Jejunum may also be used. This probably remains still the main type of urinary diversion performed following radical cystectomy.

Urinary diversion (continent)

This involves the formation of an intestinal pouch with a catheterizable cutaneous stoma. The catheterizable stoma can be constructed from ileum or appendix and is usually placed at the umbilicus or below the bikini line.

Bladder augmentation

This allows for an increase in bladder volume providing the patient with a low-capacity reservoir which may require self-catheterization to aid bladder emptying. The classical CLAM enterocystoplasty is an example of bladder augmentation. Here the bladder is bivalved and a segment of intestine or ureter can be interpositioned to bridge the defect. There are a variety of intestinal segments used which include stomach, ileum, jejunun and colon.

Bladder substitution

The bladder is replaced by the use of an intestinal segment. This is known as an orthotopic bladder substitution and means that the new bladder reservoir is anastomosed to the native urethra in a total substitution. This procedure can be performed following radical cystectomy in males and females.

In a subtotal substitution the new bladder reservoir is usually anastomosed onto the trigone and is commonly performed for more benign conditions such as interstitial cystitis.

Complications

Loss of bowel and urine contact with bowel pose the two greatest dangers. Bone disease presents a particular risk over the long term.

Continent urinary diversion is being performed with increasing frequency. Potential complications should be clear not only to clinicians who select patients and perform the surgery but also to those involved in short-term and long-term postoperative care.

Most metabolic complications result from either the bowel's contact with urine or the loss of bowel absorptive area.

Complications caused by loss of bowel

1. Gastric resection

- Reduced intrinsic factor, possibly leading to vitamin B_{12} deficiency.
- Gastric pouch ulceration.
- Theoretical risk of bone demineralization.

2. Jejunal resection

- Minimal.

3. Ileal resection

- Loss of bile acids.
- Altered lipid metabolism.
- Increased incidence of renal calculi.
- Vitamin B_{12} deficiency (terminal ileum) with potentially irreversible sequelae.
- Significant diarrhoea and malabsorptive complications (ileocaecal valve resection).

4. Colonic resection

- Diarrhoea (if ileum and right colon are resected).

Complications caused by urine contact with bowel

1. Jejunum

- Salt loss syndrome (dehydration, hyponatraemia, hypochloraemia, hyperkalaemia, metabolic acidosis).

2. Ileum

- Salt loss syndrome.
- Hyperchloraemic acidosis.

3. Colon

- Hyperchloraemic acidosis.

4. Bone disease

- Demineralization (long-term).
- Reduced growth (young patients).
- Increased fracture rate.
- Pain in weight-bearing joints.

Problems can also occur with drug absorption. This occurs as a result of drugs absorbed from the intestinal tract and excreted unmetabolized from the kidneys.

There is also an increased incidence of bacteriuria, bacteraemia and sepsis in patients that have undergone urological reconstruction using bowel segments.

The future

Since the first report on the use of bowel for augmentation cystoplasty in the late 1800s, urologists have been searching for alternative materials for bladder replacement. Bladder wall substitution has been attempted with new synthetic and organic materials; yet, a century later, intestine still remains the segment of choice. New advances in cell biology, tissue and materials sciences, and engineering, may soon change the future of bladder reconstruction. An advance over the currently proposed system of demucosalized intestinal segments for bladder augmentation may be the use of biodegradable matrices in combination with cell transplantation. Newly isolated bladder urothelial and muscle cells will attach to biodegradable polymers *in vitro* and, when implanted *in vivo*, these constructs can survive and reorganize into newly formed multi-layered structures which exhibit spatial orientation *in vivo*. The supporting matrix allows cell survival by diffusion of nutrients across short distances once a cell support matrix is implanted. The cell support matrix becomes vascularized in concert with expansion of the cell mass following implantation. These methods can be successfully employed for the *de novo* creation of functionally and anatomically normal bladders.

VARICOCELE

Varicocele is by definition an abnormal tortuous dilatation of the pampiniform plexus. Triple source of testicular arterial supply (spermatic, vasal and cremasteric arteries) is drained with a highly communicating network of veins which also function as a heat exchange mechanism to keep the testicular temperature 1–2°C below the body temperature. Pampiniform plexus drains into inferior vena cava on the right side and left renal vein on the left. Cross communications between left and right pampiniform systems has also been demonstrated.

Incidence

Approximately 5–10% of the healthy male population have varicoceles. The incidence dramatically increases over 30% among males who are treated for primary infertility. It is common on the left side and merely 5% of varicocele cases involve the right pampiniform plexus.

Grading

For clinical purposes three grades of varicocele are described:

- Grade 1: Small varicoceles that are only palpable during the Valsalva manoeuvre.
- Grade 2: Moderate size varicoceles that are palpable with the patient in a standing position.
- Grade 3: Large varicoceles that are visible through the scrotal skin and are palpable when the patient is in a standing position. Classically this grade is felt as a 'bag of worms' on palpation. Varicocele disappears at supine position and if there is a significant delay in disappearance then left renal vein obstruction due to tumour thrombus should always be excluded by further investigations.

Aetiology

There are various theories to explain the aetiology of the varicocele:

- Absent venous valves. Absent or incompetent valves of the spermatic veins have been blamed as an aetiological factor; however it has also been shown that some males have varicocele with competent venous valves or vice versa.
- Hydrostatic pressure. Pressure of the column of the blood in the left pampiniform plexus that is considerably longer than its right counterpart has been blamed as an aetiological factor.
- Nutcracker effect. The spermatic vein is compressed between aorta and superior mesenteric artery.
- An increased inflow of the arterial blood during puberty exceeding the venous drainage capacity and thus causing dilatation.

Why do we treat varicocele?

Idiopathic varicocele is asymptomatic and therefore it is either discovered during routine investigations for infertility or during medical checks such as those at school or in the army. When diagnosed at adolescence the size and the consistency of the testicle on the affected side is an important criteria for intervention.

Any delay in the normal development of the involved testicle discovered during regular ultrasound scan follow-up is an indication for treatment.

Idiopathic varicocele has long been blamed for seminal fluid analysis abnormalities. Increased incidence of varicocele among infertile man seeking treatment made it a scapegoat for abnormal seminal analysis results. Indeed some of these patients have improved qualitative and quantitative semen count after having varicocele treatment. However there is so far no controlled trial indicating that treatment of varicocele results in successful conception. In the absence of any other aetiological factor for infertility concurrent Grade 1 and Grade 2 varicoceles are a relative indication for treatment.

How do we treat varicocele?

There are currently three treatment methods available:

1. Classic surgical treatment by tying the pampiniform plexus could be performed by retroperitoneal, inguinal and scrotal approach. Success rates are highest with retroperitoneal and lowest with the scrotal approach.
2. Treatment by interventional radiologists using percutaneous approach has recently been the choice of treatment. After accessing the venous system with contralateral femoral venous puncture, leaking veins are embolized using coils and sclerosing agents. The most recent series has a success rate over 85–90% with a recurrence rate of 2–12%.
3. Laparoscopic treatment. By using this technique spermatic vessels including the spermatic artery are clipped. Testicular circulation is maintained via collateral from the artery of the vas and cremasteric artery. This method is therefore not suitable for patients who have had previous inguinal or scrotal surgery on the same side. Initial enthusiasm to treat varicoceles by laparoscopic approach is now replaced with the convenience and low morbidity of the percutaneous embolization.

VESICO-URETERIC REFLUX (VUR)

VUR is the flow of urine back from the bladder into the upper urinary tract. With increasing degrees of severity, bladder urine may reach the ureters, renal pelvis, calyces or even reflux into the collecting ducts (intrarenal reflux). VUR may be primary, meaning that there is no apparent cause, or secondary to obstruction.

Reflux nephropathy is asymmetrical renal scarring and irreversible impairment of renal function that occurs in association with persisting VUR. It is often accompanied by hypertension. VUR is present in approximately 1% of newborns, 60% of infants up to 6 months old with UTI, a third of children with UTI, and in almost all children with renal scars. Reflux nephropathy is the most common cause of end-stage renal failure in childhood.

Pathogenesis

1. Primary VUR. Normally, the ureter enters the bladder at a shallow angle so that there is a long submucosal path. During micturition, high pressure in the bladder compresses the intramural portion of the ureter against the firmly contracting bladder wall and prevents reflux of urine. In primary VUR, the ureter enters more nearly perpendicular to the bladder wall and the anti-reflux mechanism is less efficient; as the detrusor contracts, urine is forced back into the ureter. VUR is familial in a third of cases. As a child grows and the bladder enlarges, the course of the ureter becomes more oblique and reflux may lessen or disappear.

2. Secondary VUR. Reflux is common in those with congenital urinary obstruction or neurogenic bladder from spinal cord injury.

Pathophysiology

If reflux is sufficiently severe, retrograde flow of urine into the collecting ducts incites an inflammatory reaction and initiates events that culminate in reflux nephropathy. The exact pathogenic mechanisms of reflux nephropathy are disputed. Damage appears to result partly from congenital hypoplasia and partly from acquired scarring. Possibly forcible intrusion of distal tubular urine containing Tamm–Horsfall protein into the medullary interstitium causes inflammation. Inflammation proceeds to renal scarring and interstitial fibrosis, most marked in the renal medulla, but also extending into the cortex. Scarring is often accompanied by hypertension.

Another mechanism, in only a few patients, is the development of a secondary glomerular lesion (focal segmental glomerulosclerosis). This shows itself as proteinuria and then almost inevitable progression to end-stage renal disease. The mechanism is unknown but it may represent 'overload nephropathy' from loss of nephrons through scarring.

The role of urinary tract infection (UTI) in the genesis of reflux nephropathy is uncertain. It may worsen scarring and interstitial inflammation, and UTI can be difficult to eradicate in the presence of reflux. End-stage renal disease occurs in patients who have never had a UTI.

Clinical features

VUR is usually silent. Most cases come to light because of UTI. This is most common in infancy, and the high probability of finding VUR is the reason for imaging the urinary tract in all infants with a UTI.

A few patients will first present with hypertension, nocturnal enuresis, protein-uria, or with other urologic problems. Some are not detected until they present with advanced renal failure, commonly in the late teens or early adult life.

Diagnosis

Imaging of the kidney (in various ways, but sonogram is a good way to start) may show depressed cortical scars overlying dilated ('clubbed') calyces. Only 25% of children have hydronephrosis, therefore it is important to perform a voiding cysto-urethrogram. Voiding cysto-urethrogram (VCUG) will demonstrate the reflux. Diagnosis of reflux nephropathy may be difficult if there has been damage from prior reflux, but reflux is no longer present when the VCUG is done.

Vesico-ureteric grading

Numerous grading systems are described but the most widely accepted is the International System. This has five grades. The distribution of grades are shown in parentheses. Approximately half of affected children have bilateral reflux.

Grade 1: The contrast enters the ureter but does not enter the renal pelvis (5–8%).
Grade 2: The contrast material reaches the pelvis but does not distend the collecting system (35%).
Grade 3: The collecting system is filled and either the ureter or pelvis is distended but the calyceal demarcations are not distorted (25–35%).
Grade 4: The dilated ureter is slightly tortuous and the calyces are blunted significantly (15–25%).
Grade 5: The entire collecting system is tremendously dilated without a visible papillary impression, and there is significant ureteral tortuosity (5%).

Management

The management of this condition still remains very controversial. The important factors are to detect urinary tract infections promptly, and treat with adequate courses of antibiotics. The eradication of infection by repeat culture 3 days after the end of antibiotics is performed with the overall aim to keep the urine sterile.

Surgical re-implantation of the ureters into the bladder can stop reflux. It has a place in severe reflux in the first 2–3 years of life. Surgery, however, does not affect progression to renal failure and surgery does not affect incidence of UTI. It may help, however, in occasional severe cases. Endoscopic therapies, including Submucosal Teflon Injection (STING), have been used, but because of emboliza-tion risks from this material, bioplastique or collagen are now routinely used. This is inferior to open surgery, but has a success of about 70% with one procedure. Repeat submucosal injection procedures do have a cure rate of up to 90–95%.

Further reading

Lewitt SB. Medical versus surgical treatment of primary vesicoureteral reflux: report of the international reflux study committee. *Paediatrics*, 1981; **67**: 392.

INDEX

The KEY TOPICS Series

Advisors:

T.M. Craft *Department of Anaesthesia and Intensive Care, Royal United Hospital, Bath, UK*
C.S. Garrard *Intensive Therapy Unit, John Radcliffe Hospital, Oxford, UK*
P.M. Upton *Department of Anaesthesia, Royal Cornwall Hospital, Treliske, Truro, UK*

Accident and Emergency Medicine, Second Edition
Anaesthesia – Clinical Aspects, Third Edition
Cardiovascular Medicine
Chronic Pain, Second Edition
Critical Care
Evidence-Based Medicine
Gastroenterology
General Surgery, Second Edition
Neonatology
Neurology
Obstetrics and Gynaecology, Second Edition
Oncology
Ophthalmology, Second Edition
Oral and Maxillofacial Surgery
Orthopaedic Surgery
Orthopaedic Trauma Surgery
Otolaryngology, Second Edition
Paediatrics, Second Edition
Psychiatry
Renal Medicine
Respiratory Medicine
Thoracic Surgery
Trauma

Forthcoming titles include:

Acute Poisoning
Cardiac Surgery
Clinical Research

UROLOGY